TALKING WITH COLLEGE STUDENTS
ABOUT ALCOHOL

TALKING with COLLEGE STUDENTS about ALCOHOL

MOTIVATIONAL STRATEGIES FOR REDUCING ABUSE

Scott T. Walters
John S. Baer

THE GUILFORD PRESS
New York   London

To our wives, Kelli Walters and Margaret Carney,
who encourage us by their example to be better listeners
and speakers

Library of Congress Cataloging-in-Publication Data

Walters, Scott T.
    Talking with college students about alcohol: motivational strategies for reducing abuse / Scott T. Walters, John S. Baer.
        p. cm.
    Includes bibliographical references and index.
    ISBN 1-59385-222-3 (pbk.: alk. paper)
1. College students—Alcohol use—United States—Prevention.   I. Baer, John Samuel, 1958–   II. Title.
    HV5135.W36 2006
    362.292′86—dc22

                                                              2005020981

About the Authors

Scott T. Walters, PhD, is Assistant Professor of Behavioral Sciences at the University of Texas School of Public Health. His research interests include college student health and substance abuse prevention, brief negotiation in medical settings, and religious/spiritual aspects of psychology. He has written more than 30 articles and book chapters on theoretical and applied aspects of psychology as well as two books for children. He is also coeditor of the book *Treating Substance Abuse: Theory and Technique.* Dr. Walters acts as a consultant for several treatment agencies; is a frequent speaker to campus, community, and medical groups; and has received national and international awards for his work.

John S. Baer, PhD, is Research Associate Professor in the Department of Psychology at the University of Washington in Seattle, and is also Associate Director for Training and Education at the Center of Excellence for Substance Abuse Treatment and Education at the VA Puget Sound Health Care System. Dr. Baer's research and clinical interests focus on the assessment, prevention, treatment, and relapse of substance use and abuse. He has specialized in the study of brief interventions for both prevention and treatment, and has recently begun research on professional training in motivational interviewing. Dr. Baer has provided workshops on substance abuse, relapse prevention, early intervention for problem drinking, and motivational interviewing for over 15 years. He also maintains a small private clinical practice.

Preface

Through pictures, testimonials, and heart-wrenching stories, the media have recently chronicled the problem of college drinking. This new focus has brought to general attention something alcohol researchers and many college graduates have known since the 1950s: Heavy drinking is common on college campuses and is associated with a host of social and personal problems. In response, government reports and the popular press have made recommendations for colleges seeking to reduce drinking and its associated consequences. These recommendations have included changes in alcohol availability and pricing, advertising, and a range of policies that cover class meeting times, penalties for alcohol use, parental notification, and regulation of social organizations. In addition, educators and psychologists have described a panoply of prevention and intervention programs, ranging from mass marketing campaigns aimed at the entire student body to clinical protocols for students who are already having difficulties.

Unfortunately, policy recommendations and prevention programs offer little direction for those who interact with students individually or in small groups. At the same time, many clinical intervention protocols have not been disseminated effectively. Some interventions remain cloistered in academic research journals, while others require significant modifications to be used in everyday practice. Interventions tested in research settings may assume a relatively sophisticated knowledge of college student development and counseling, require questionnaires and procedures that are too lengthy to be used in most settings, and be too rigid in the way they are supposed to be implemented.

Yet studies suggest that there are several brief and effective behavior change interventions that can be conducted, even by people with relatively little specialized training. Effective programs range from personalized feedback delivered through the mail to 50-minute interventions delivered by college peers. In other contexts, even 5-minute interactions in medical settings or over the phone have shown lasting effects. This new emphasis on brevity, flexibility, and delivery by nonspecialists represents an opportunity to expand the utilization of effective methods.

We wrote this book not because we developed a new therapy for college drinking, but because we wanted to make existing approaches easier to use. This book is meant to be a practical guide for those who talk with students about alcohol, especially "frontline" professionals, such as counselors, health educators, psychologists, physicians, and other student health and service personnel. In making recommendations, we have attempted to balance what we know as clinicians and researchers with our experience as trainers of counselors, health personnel, and educators. We understand that college prevention workers have many constraints in their work—real limits in the way they can screen and intervene with students in increasingly brief and sometimes chaotic settings. We are also keenly aware that the translation of research protocols into day-to-day practice requires a good deal of flexibility. Thus, drawing from the literature on college student development, motivational counseling, skills training, and brief negotiation in medical settings, we provide several options for interacting with students, depending on available time and resources. Balancing scientific rigor on the one hand and flexibility in application on the other hand is not easy. Science can be quite helpful in selecting prevention or treatment approaches, and we have endeavored to recommend empirically supported approaches. At the same time we admit that the scientific base for college drinking interventions is still rather limited. Thus, we have made recommendations using our knowledge of research, clinical experience, and, in some cases, our best guess. Our hope is that these strategies will fall into the hands of those who need them the most and ultimately become a larger part of the effort to encourage students and communities toward greater health and safety.

This book is divided into three rough sections. The first group of chapters is focused on how and why college students drink. Chapter 1 sets the stage by discussing "what" questions. How bad is the problem? Has it gotten better or worse? Chapter 2 approaches the "why" and "how" questions. Why do college students drink? How do conversations about alcohol fit into the larger picture? The way we understand the issues related to college drinking largely determines the approach we take to remedying the problem. Thus, in this first section, we provide answers to some of these important questions as a way to frame the suggestions we make in later chapters.

The second group of chapters provides information about assessment and counseling style. Chapter 3 discusses practical ways to assess and use information about drinking and related areas. Chapter 4 discusses the spirit and style of motivational interviewing (MI), an evidence-based counseling style for promoting behavior change. The MI approach is fundamental to the strategies we detail in later chapters.

The third group of chapters covers specific types of interactions. We divide our suggestions roughly based on available time. If you have 5–10 minutes with a student, Chapter 5 makes recommendations for providing brief advice. There is some evidence that these ultra-brief encounters reduce drinking, particularly when delivered in a healthcare setting. If you have 10–30 minutes with a student, we recommend what we call a behavioral consultation. Also described in Chapter 5, behavioral consultations expand on brief advice through increased use of MI and the use of a few simple motivational techniques. If you have 30–50 minutes with a student, we recommend the motivational intervention described in Chapter 6. This intervention perhaps has the greatest empirical support and makes full use of the MI principles described in Chapter 4. This intervention also includes personalized feedback, a relatively easy way to structure a longer interaction. If you have more than 50 minutes, or have multiple interactions with a student, Chapter 6 presents additional activities that can be helpful. In Chapter 7, we describe how to use MI principles with groups of students, and provide an example of a one- to three-session motivational group. Chapter 8 provides suggestions for integrating individual or group conversation into the larger treatment system and campus community. Finally, the appendices contain a number of reproducible assessments, questionnaires, and handouts to implement the interventions more easily.

Although we have tried to assemble them as coherent, self-contained interactions, we are aware that conversations about alcohol come in many shapes and sizes. Nurses and doctors may have, by necessity, different goals and constraints than college counselors. Each provider should choose the approach (or approaches) that makes the most sense given his or her contact with students. Likewise, we encourage the reader to add or subtract elements from these interventions as appropriate. We hope the material in this book will support those who work in college health, residence life, and other student service settings. Not all students drink in a heavy or dangerous fashion, but for those who do, there are effective strategies to promote contemplation, motivation, and risk reduction.

Acknowledgments

A number of individuals helped to form this book. First and foremost, we owe a great debt, both personally and professionally, to William Miller and Stephen Rollnick, the developers of the motivational interviewing (MI) approach. Also influential in our thinking have been colleagues at the University of Washington who have focused so effectively on problems with college drinking. We greatly appreciate the contributions of the coauthors of the original BASICS curriculum, and those who have published and trained using motivational models, including G. Alan Marlatt, Dan Kivlahan, Linda Dimeff, Mary Larimer, Jason Kilmer, and George Parks. We also thank the number of authors of clinical handbooks whose ideas and techniques we adapted in this book. We have attempted to acknowledge these individuals directly in the text.

We also acknowledge the many informal contributions of the Motivational Interviewing Network of Trainers (affectionately known as the "Minties"). Through annual meetings, videotapes, newsletters, and listserv conversations, the interactions with this group shaped our thinking about how to present this material. In particular, David Rosengren and Chris Dunn have generously shared their expertise and been exemplary models of MI training.

Amanda Matson provided tireless assistance with BAC tables and referencing. Other colleagues in Dallas and Seattle supported this effort with thoughtful feedback and by affording us tremendous academic freedom.

Kitty Moore and Jim Nageotte, at The Guilford Press, provided shepherding and editorial advice on our manuscript. They were calm and thoughtful voices throughout our sometimes scattered process of writing. Our team of "practice" editors—Betsy Foy, Jennifer Rykard, and Bob Schroeder—and three additional anonymous editors read the entire in-progress manuscript, and provided a number of helpful suggestions on how to best tailor the book to our readership. Their collective experience in the field added immeasurably to the final product.

Those we have trained, of course, have shaped us to a great extent. Indeed, much of this book is in response to questions and needs that have arisen when we have tried to help college practitioners adapt programs to their campuses. Smart and penetrating questions have forced us to modify and tailor programs to meet the real needs of those who talk with college students on a daily basis.

Finally, we acknowledge the large contribution that college students have made over the years to our understanding of young adult drinking. Their willingness to speak honestly about their alcohol use, to pose difficult questions, and to provide us with feedback on our methods has changed our conversations for the better.

Contents

1. WHAT'S HAPPENING ON CAMPUS?   1

Overview of the Chapter 1
Rates of Drinking   1
Perceptions and Misperceptions   4
Drinking-Related Consequences   8
What Isn't Said   9
What Students Think about Drinking and Getting Drunk   10
Managing the Disconnect   11
Key Points   12

2. RESPONDING TO COLLEGE DRINKING   13

Overview of the Chapter   13
Models of Alcohol Problems   13
College Students and Risk   14
Drinking and Development   16
When Change Occurs   17
Implications for Intervention   19
What Works in Prevention and Treatment?   20
How This Book Fits In   21
Organizing the Toolbox   23
Key Points   24

3. ASSESSING DRINKING AND RELATED BEHAVIORS   25

Overview of the Chapter   25
When and Where to Assess Drinking   26
Alcohol Consumption   27
Alcohol Screening   35
Related Areas   36
Conclusion   39
Key Points   41

4. STYLE OF THE INTERACTION   42

Overview of the Chapter   42
Who Can Talk to Students about Alcohol?   43
Deconstructing the Style of the Interview   43
Working with Motivation   44
Core Techniques   48
What Comes Next?   59
Key Points   59

5. BRIEF INDIVIDUAL INTERACTIONS: ADVICE AND CONSULTATION   60

Overview of the Chapter   60
What Motivates People in Brief Interactions?   61
Broaching the Subject   61
Providing Advice and Suggestions   63
Exploring Change in the Abstract   66
Importance and Confidence Rulers   67
Closing the Interaction   70
Sample Brief Advice (3–10 Minutes)   71
Sample Behavioral Consultation (10–30 Minutes)   72
Key Points   73

6. EXTENDED INDIVIDUAL INTERACTIONS   75

Overview of the Chapter   75
Opening and Closing Longer Interactions   76
Talking about Change (When It Makes Sense to Do So)   80
Motivational Exercises   83
Sample Motivational Intervention (Four Sessions, 60 Minutes Each)   95
Key Points   100

7. TALKING WITH COLLEGE DRINKERS IN A GROUP   101

Overview of the Chapter   101
Rationale and Challenges of Group Programs   102
Structure and Spirit of the Good Group   104
Strategies for Groups   113
Sample Group Intervention (120–180 Minutes, over One to Three Sessions)   120
Key Points   122

8. SERVICE INTEGRATION AND TRAINING   123

Overview of the Chapter   123
How Students Receive Services   123
Integrating Services   125
Delivering Services and Following Up   127
Training and Evaluation   128
Final Comment   130
Key Points   131

APPENDICES   133

Measures   135
Clinical Exercises and Materials   156

REFERENCES   201

INDEX   209

1

What's Happening on Campus?

OVERVIEW OF THE CHAPTER

College students drink. No matter how you slice it, most people would agree with some version of that statement. But what do the words mean? That *all* students drink? That students drink heavily or frequently? That it is normal for young adults to drink to intoxication? That alcohol creates big problems?

College drinking can clearly be excessive and dangerous. Yet, how we answer these questions depends on what information we think is important, what we think should be "normal" for young people, and how we understand the context in which college drinking occurs. There are certainly myths and misinformation about drinking during college, and we believe these myths result in less productive prevention and treatment efforts. Conversely, accurate information helps us not only to design effective prevention and treatment programs, but also to communicate with students directly. Because of this, we begin by discussing rates, perceptions, and problems related to college drinking.

RATES OF DRINKING

Drinking is typically measured in two ways: *frequency*—how often a person drinks—and *quantity*—how much is consumed when a person drinks. In standard clinical parlance, frequency refers to the number of days a student consumed any alcohol over the last week or month. To make drinks equivalent, quantity is usually measured in "standard" drinks. In the United States, one standard drink = half an ounce of ethanol, roughly the amount of alcohol in a 12-ounce beer, 4 ounces of wine, or 1¼ ounces of 80-proof spirits. Multiplying quantity and frequency gets an average number over a period, for instance *drinks per week* or *month*.

Although quantity and frequency averages are often used to describe drinking, they can mask important distinctions when it comes to health and safety risk. For example, one individual might consume 12 drinks per week over four different occasions, while another might consume 12 drinks all on one night. Due to the greater risk for intoxication, accidents, health effects, and social consequences, the latter pattern (i.e., 12 all at once) is more worrisome. Because of this, a different measure is sometimes useful. *Episodic heavy drinking*—sometimes called a "binge" episode[1]—is the consumption of a large amount of alcohol in a short amount of time.[2] The most commonly used threshold is five or more drinks in a row. (Because of the size and metabolic differences between males and females, some studies use five or more for men and four or more for women.) The frequency of heavy-drinking episodes is a good indicator of risky drinking among college students.

With these measures in mind, O'Malley and Johnston (2002) recently summarized the results of five large U.S. surveys. Sources included the College Alcohol Studies (CAS; Wechsler, Dowdall, Maenner, Gledhill-Hoyt, & Lee, 1998; www.hsph.harvard.edu/cas), the CORE Institute studies (CORE; Presley, Meilman, Cashin, & Lyerla, 1996; www.siu.edu/~coreinst), the Monitoring the Future studies (MTF; Johnston, O'Malley, & Bachman, 2001, 2002; www.monitoringthefuture.org), the National College Health Risk Behavior Survey (NCHRBS; Centers for Disease Control and Prevention; www.cdc.gov/epo/mmwr/preview/mmwrhtml/00049859.htm), and the National Household Survey on Drug Abuse (NHSDA; U.S. Substance Abuse and Mental Health Services Administration; Gfroerer, Greenblatt, & Wright, 1997; www.samhsa.gov). Drawing on aggregate data, O'Malley and Johnston concluded that, on average, 65–70% of U.S. college students reported some alcohol consumption in the 30 days prior to the survey. In terms of heavy drinking, as shown in Figure 1.1, 40–44% of students reported consuming five or more drinks in a single episode during the previous month. This means that approximately two-thirds of students drink some alcohol in a given month, and more than half of drinkers report at least one heavy episode. Finally, within this group of heavy episodic drinkers, there is a smaller number that reports *frequent* heavy episodes. Not all surveys report this metric, but those that do (e.g., Wechsler, Molnar, Davenport, & Baer, 1999) find that less than half of heavy drinkers—about 17–19% of all students—drink heavily *and* frequently (two to three times a week or more). Daily drinking, however, is relatively rare among college students, with most surveys reporting about a 5% incidence rate.

Among the demographic variables related to drinking, gender is the best predictor; across the board, men drink more, and more often, than women do (O'Malley & Johnston, 2002). This pattern is clearly visible in Figure 1.1. Part of the reason for this is that men are larger and have more fluid relative to body weight than women, but corrections for body

---

[1]There has been great controversy over the use of "binge" to describe college student drinking. We agree with DeJong (2001) that this threshold is somewhat arbitrary and that the term "binge" probably reinforces an exaggerated view of student drinking. We prefer the more neutral term *episodic heavy drinking*.

[2]In February 2004, the National Institute on Alcohol Abuse and Alcoholism (NIAAA) National Advisory Council suggested that a "binge" be used to describe an episode of five or more drinks for men or four or more drinks for women *within a period of about two hours*. Most surveys, though, have not used such a discrete time period.

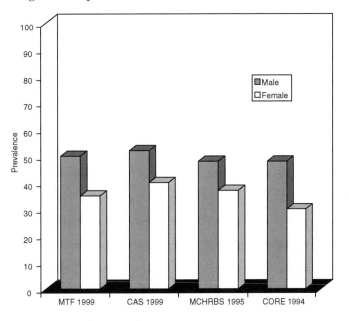

FIGURE 1.1. Prevalence of heavy drinking among college students, by gender. From O'Malley and Johnston (2002). Reprinted with permission from *Journal of Studies on Alcohol*, Supplement No. 14, pp. 23–39, 2002. Copyright by Alcohol Research Documentation, Inc., Rutgers Center of Alcohol Studies, Piscataway, NJ 08854.

size do not completely eliminate the gender difference. The gap may be closing, but for now, it remains a robust finding—about 50% of college men and 37% of college women report a heavy-drinking episode in the past month.

Of course, one should be careful of averages. When surveys ask students how much and how often they drink, they usually provide categories for answers (e.g., zero times per week, one to two times a week, three to four times a week), but these categories may not reflect the way students actually drink. Other studies support a more nuanced view of college drinking. For example, Del Boca, Darkes, Greenbaum, and Goldman (2004) asked college students to keep daily logs of drinking over an entire academic year. The diaries showed that students did drink heavily on occasion. However, the occasions tended to vary, not with time (e.g., every weekend), but with *event* (e.g., holidays, celebrations, football games). Moreover, students usually did *not* drink near events that required their full and sober attention, such as final papers and end-of-term exams. This means that, rather than being a daily or weekly aspect of campus life, alcohol consumption is more often variable and opportunistic. Another recent study took random alcohol breath analyses of students returning to their dormitories at night (Thombs, Olds, & Snyder, 2003). Roughly half had consumed alcohol, but most had quite moderate alcohol readings. Even those who reported consuming five or more drinks that evening, for the most part did not have alcohol readings in the intoxicated range. Although this study examined students at only one university, it suggests that asking students whether they consumed five or more drinks in one sitting may overrepresent rates of intoxication.

PERCEPTIONS AND MISPERCEPTIONS

A few key issues shape the way we understand and respond to college drinking. For instance, has college drinking gotten worse or better? Do college students drink more than other young people? Do some colleges have higher rates of drinking than others? The answers to these questions—correct or not—determine what attention the problem gets, what programs get funded, and ultimately what we say to students about drinking.

Is heavy drinking specific to college students, or is it a general finding among young people? The answer seems to be both. O'Malley and Johnston (2002) reviewed two large data sets that compared young adults in college to their same-age peers not in college. In all comparisons, college students drank more frequently and in greater quantities than those not enrolled in college. The surveys also showed that young adults tended to increase their drinking dramatically upon entrance of college. This is ironic given that, when in high school, college-bound students drank significantly *less* than their non-college-bound peers (Figure 1.2). Both groups of students tended to increase their drinking after graduating from high school, but students who went on to college increased significantly more and actually surpassed their non-college student peers. A recent study by

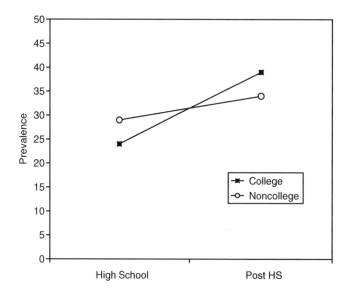

FIGURE 1.2. Change in heavy drinking from high school senior year to post high school (MTF 1997–1999 data combined). From O'Malley and Johnston (2002). Reprinted with permission from *Journal of Studies on Alcohol*, Supplement No. 14, pp. 23–39, 2002. Copyright by Alcohol Research Documentation, Inc., Rutgers Center of Alcohol Studies, Piscataway, NJ 08854.

Slutske and colleagues (Slutske et al., 2004) provides even more information about this pattern for college women. This group of researchers examined differences in drinking practices between college and non-college females while taking into account differences in demographics, lifestyle factors, and family background. While all these background measures were associated with drinking, they could not account for one specific difference between those who were and were not in college: occasional heavy drinking. In other words, heavy episodic drinking was specifically associated with college attendance.

In fairness, it is important to note that the differences between college and non-college groups are relatively small and the overall patterns of consumption relatively similar. For example, in the MTF study (Johnston et al., 2001), 41% of college students reported heavy drinking in the past two weeks, whereas 37% of non-college individuals did so. Thus, there does seem to be something about the college culture that promotes heavy drinking, even though the pattern is relatively common in this age group.

Does heavy drinking vary from college to college? Yes. Weschler and colleagues (1999) report a wide range of drinking rates across U.S. colleges. In this survey, rates of heavy drinking varied from 10 to 65%, depending on the institution. Several factors seem to contribute to this intercampus variability, though none completely explains the difference (Presley, Meilman, & Leichliter, 2002). First, drinking varies with region. Colleges in the Northeast have the highest heavy-drinking rates, followed by schools in the north-central and western states. Southern schools have the lowest rates. Second, colleges with higher rates of heavy drinking usually have a greater proportion of male students, greater memberships in fraternities and sororities, a younger student body, more students living on campus, and a greater proportion of white students. (Minority students tend to drink less than Caucasian students.) Finally, the literature suggests that community norms are linked to drinking rates. As evidenced by the infamous *Princeton Review* and *Playboy* surveys, there clearly are "party" schools, and their reputations as such may perpetuate drinking practices more strongly than any regional or demographic factors.

How different is college drinking from older adult drinking? The answer may be surprising. On the one hand, heavy drinking tends to decline over time. From the MTF surveys (Johnston et al., 2001), we know that heavy episodic drinking peaks at 42% around ages 21–22, and then steadily declines to about 24% by ages 31–32 (see Figure 1.3). The vast majority of college students greatly reduce their heavy drinking once they leave college (Jessor, Donovan, & Costa, 1991; Baer, MacLean, & Marlatt, 1998). However, unlike heavy *episodic* drinking, rates of *daily* drinking do not decline, sticking at about 5% throughout the 20s. Then again, even adults drink heavily at times. As shown in Figure 1.3, when Johnston and colleagues (2001) followed individuals into middle adulthood, they found that at age 40, 26% still reported at least one heavy episode during the past two weeks. In a similar way, Naimi and colleagues (2003) used data from the Behavioral Risk Factor Surveillance System (BRFSS), a multistate telephone survey of over 200,000 people, to examine heavy drinking in the U.S. population. Consistent with MTF data, BRFSS data show that, although rates of heavy drinking were highest among those ages 18–26, those who were older than 26 accounted for 69% of heavy-drinking episodes. Moreover,

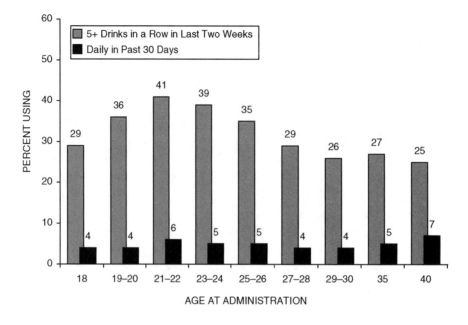

FIGURE 1.3. Two-week prevalence of daily and heavy episodic drinking, ages 18–40 (Johnston et al., 2002).

Naimi and colleagues (2003) report that 73% of heavy episodes occurred among people who were otherwise moderate drinkers. Our point is that heavy drinking and its associated risks are found throughout the U.S. population, not only among young people and not only among those with chronic drinking patterns.

Has heavy drinking gotten worse in recent years? The answer to this question is not clear, as different surveys report different trends (see Figure 1.4). Naimi and colleagues (2003), using BRFSS data, found that rates of heavy drinking among 18- to 20-year-olds increased slightly, from 23% in 1993 to 26.1% in 2001. In contrast, the MTF studies suggest that heavy drinking by young people has decreased over the past 20 years, from 45% in 1984 to 40% in 1999 (O'Malley & Johnston, 2002). Interestingly, Wechsler and colleagues (2002) report a polarization of drinking patterns over the 1990s, with greater rates of both abstinence and frequent heavy drinking. In sum, recent data are mixed and may indicate either increased or decreased heavy drinking, depending on which study you look at.

In terms of long-term changes, we can compare recent college data to the seminal 1953 survey conducted by Robert Straus and Seldon Bacon. Straus and Bacon actually completed an excellent survey by today's standards. They surveyed 17,000 students at 27 institutions that were selected to represent a range of demographic features, including small colleges and large universities, urban and rural settings, private and public funding, and colleges with students of different races. O'Malley and Johnston (2002) compare the monthly prevalence of 65% from Straus and Bacon in 1953 with recent MTF and CAS estimates of 68% and 70% and conclude that drinking has indeed increased slightly over the last 50 years. In addition, as O'Malley and Johnston (2002) note, the demography of college students has changed since the 1950s, in particular with a much higher percentage of women and minorities attending college. Given that white men, on average, drink more than men of other racial groups and women, this probably means that there has been a larger increase within groups than simple averages might suggest. Comparing Straus and Bacon's measures of *heavy* drinking to today's (unfortunately, the measures are somewhat different) suggests a modest 50-year increase in rates for men and a more substantial increase for women.

In sum, alcohol use during college, and specifically heavy episodic drinking, has a long cultural history in the United States. Rates among men have increased slightly over the last 50 years, while rates among women have increased substantially. Over the past 20 years, though, patterns appear to be more stable. Rates also seem to be associated with certain cultural, regional, and environmental factors, which may reinforce or discourage certain practices. Drinking, and occasional heavy drinking, is relatively common among all ages, including young people not enrolled in college.

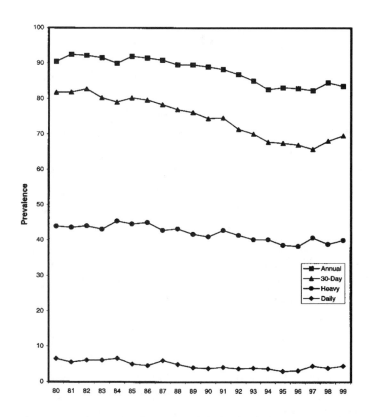

FIGURE 1.4. Trends in annual, 30-day, heavy, and daily drinking among college students, 1980–1999. From O'Malley and Johnston (2002). Reprinted with permission from *Journal of Studies on Alcohol*, Supplement No. 14, pp. 23–39, 2002. Copyright by Alcohol Research Documentation, Inc., Rutgers Center of Alcohol Studies, Piscataway, NJ 08854.

What about other drug use? Students use substances other than alcohol, but much less commonly. After alcohol, tobacco and marijuana are the drugs of choice. In the same national surveys mentioned earlier, almost a third of college students reported smoking cigarettes in the past 30 days and about 20% reported using marijuana, though rates of *daily* use of these substances were considerably lower (O'Malley & Johnston, 2002). Less than 2% of students reported current use of cocaine. Interestingly, college students use *less* cocaine, marijuana, and tobacco than do their non-college peers—a pattern opposite that of alcohol. Thus, while the college culture may promote risky drinking, it does not seem to promote drug use in the same way.

In this book, we focus on alcohol because of the preponderance of problems it creates on college campuses. In taking this narrow focus, we recognize that we have sidestepped many of the issues that appear with real-life students. Students often have concerns or difficulties with substances other than, or in addition to, alcohol. Despite this limitation, we believe that many of the counseling strategies we recommend can be helpful in talking with college students about other drugs abused (or behavior change more generally). We encourage providers to generalize these models.

DRINKING-RELATED CONSEQUENCES

Students who drink heavily and frequently have more accidents, are involved more frequently in violent activities, do worse in college, and generally make life more difficult for those who live around them than students who do not (Perkins, 2002). While it would be naive to suggest that if alcohol were eliminated from college life, all health and safety problems would disappear, alcohol is clearly associated with many difficulties. The most obvious consequences of alcohol use are the well-publicized injuries and deaths. On average, about 10% of students report physical injuries in the last year as a result of drinking (Wechsler et al., 1998; Presley et al., 1996). Rates of intoxicated driving are also high. Engs, Diebold, and Hansen (1996) found that 56% of male heavy drinkers and 43% of female heavy drinkers had likely driven drunk in the previous year. Hingson, Heeren, Zakocs, Kopstein, and Wechsler (2002), using data from the National Highway Transportation Safety Administration and other surveys, estimate that 1,400 college students died in 1998 as a result of alcohol-related injuries and traffic accidents.

In addition to injuries and traffic fatalities, alcohol itself can be fatal if consumed in large-enough quantities. We are unaware of systematic data on rates of alcohol poisoning on college campuses, but employees of university health centers and nearby emergency rooms can attest to its occurrence. Alcohol consumption is also associated with greater sexual risks. Many students use alcohol to meet and be sexual with others, and for some, alcohol is associated with unplanned, unprotected, or aggressive sex (Perkins, 2002). For instance, in one large, anonymous survey, 12% of male drinkers and 4% of female drinkers admitted taking advantage of someone sexually through alcohol or drug use (Presley et al., 1996). In another survey, nearly half of students reported that drinking had gotten them in sexual situations they later regretted (Larimer, Lydum, Anderson, & Turner, 1999).

Alcohol consumption is also associated with worse academic performance. Heavy episodic drinkers do worse on tests, miss more classes, and have lower grade point averages (GPA) than other students (Perkins, 2002). Although alcohol use is correlated with GPA (i.e., on average, higher use = lower grades), at least one study suggests that the role of alcohol may not be causal and that other factors may cause both drinking and lower grades (Wood, Sher, Erickson, & DeBord, 1997).

Finally, college-student drinking creates problems for others (Perkins, 2002). In addition to the risk of sexual assault noted above, drinking is related to property damage, vandalism, and physical fights. In one study, 30% of students reported getting into a fight in the past year because of drinking (Presley et al., 1996). Wechsler, Moeykens, Davenport, Castillo, and Hansen (1995) have also shown that nearly half of all students (43%) experienced interruptions in their studies or sleep because of another's alcohol consumption. This substantial secondhand cost to institutions and communities includes reparation of damage, adjudication of students who violate rules, medical costs, security, and prevention and counseling services.

WHAT ISN'T SAID

The patterns and consequences of drinking common in American universities should raise alarm. Administrators, teachers, health professionals, parents, and students are right in wanting to reduce the harms associated with drinking. However, we must be careful not to sensationalize campus drinking, as some in the media have done through splashy pictures of out-of-control, lascivious, or rioting students. For most students, the pictures don't fit. First, as is clear from the data presented above, not every college student drinks or drinks heavily. In fact, almost a third of college students report not drinking at all in the past month, and many others drink quite moderately. Second, not all students who drink heavily do so frequently, and many of these occasional heavy drinkers report no negative experiences as a result. When Wechsler and colleagues (1999) divided students into those who drank heavily *occasionally* and those who drank heavily *frequently*, they found that the greatest harm was attributable to the 19% of students who drank heavily *and* frequently. In fact, these 19% of students accounted for 68% of all the alcohol consumed *by the entire sample*. Thus, while this 19% figure is higher than we would like, it is nevertheless much smaller than the 43% binge drinking figure sometimes promulgated by the media. Furthermore, considering that people of all age groups sometimes drink to intoxication, this means that about 80% of college students drink in a way that is consistent with the larger U.S. culture. Finally, one drinking consequence that is usually not found among college students is alcohol dependence. As defined by the American Psychiatric Association (DSM-IV; American Psychiatric Association, 1994), alcohol dependence is a cluster of physiological, psychological, and social problems related to alcohol use (see Chapter 3). Research by Knight and colleagues (2002) suggests that 6.3% of college students endorse enough symptoms over the past year to warrant a formal diagnosis of alcohol dependence. This figure alone is clearly cause for concern. However, for the most part, college students are young and healthy, have good social connections, and drink—if they drink—opportunistically. In addition, longitudinal data clearly show that most college drinkers will outgrow these patterns once they leave college and enter the workforce (Jessor et al., 1991; Sher, Bartholow, & Nanda, 2001). Heavy drinking in college, for the most part, does not lead to chronic problems in later life.

WHAT STUDENTS THINK ABOUT DRINKING AND GETTING DRUNK

The data we have presented thus far come from large surveys of college drinking and observations by college administrators, faculty, and health professionals. One important consideration remains: What do *students* think about drinking? Although students have many perspectives, one finding is rather consistent: In general, college students are much less concerned about alcohol than older members of the community. Because of this, students are likewise not clamoring for alcohol-prevention programs. In our own research, we have sometimes joked that it was hard to get students to attend a program if the words "alcohol" and "education" were both in the title. Rather, students routinely groan when told that alcohol use is dangerous or against the rules. Many feel that they have learned all they need to know about alcohol in high school health classes or from parents. In fact, after one program, one of us (JSB) was told that the material he was presenting would be better for younger participants. Seniors in the audience felt it would be better for freshman, and freshman thought it would be better for high school seniors. Everyone thought it would be better for someone else.

There are several reasons college students are, in general, less concerned about drinking. First, young people tend to use more liberal criteria in defining drinking-related problems. Posavac (1993) asked students if certain behaviors constituted a "problem" with alcohol. As long as they did not occur frequently, most students were unwilling to label vomiting, missed classes, fights, and blackouts as problems. Second, students tend to misperceive drinking norms on campus, believing that other students drink more and experience more alcohol-related problems than they actually do (Baer, Stacy, & Larimer, 1991; Kypri & Langley, 2003) and that others are more accepting of heavy drinking than they actually are (Perkins & Berkowitz, 1986). In one study, only 9% of respondents thought that they drank more than the average student at their university (Kypri & Langley, 2003). Third, consistent with social psychology research, students tend to think *others* are more at risk for alcohol-related problems than they are and view their own behavior as situation specific, as compared to others' behavior, which they saw as more permanent or fixed. In at least one study, college students were more likely to define an alcohol-related consequence as a problem for others than they were for themselves (Baer & Carney, 1993). Finally, like other adult drinkers, college students expect alcohol to produce a series of positive effects—relaxation, socialization, sexuality—and the strength of these positive expectancies is related to drinking (Carey & Correia, 1997; Goldman, Greenbaum, & Darkes, 1997; Neighbors, Walker, & Larimer, 2003).

Perhaps most obviously, college drinking is a social behavior. Social organizations, such as fraternities, sororities, athletic teams, and even academic groups, have well-established drinking practices and customs. Alcohol is commonly consumed in social situations where males and females meet and date, as well as before, during, and after athletic events (Nelson & Wechsler, 2003). Students even rate heavy-drinking fraternities as being of higher social status (Larimer, Irvine, Kilmer, & Marlatt, 1997). Thus, far from being seen as an evil influence, alcohol is typically perceived as a positive social force and a normal part of college life.

This is not to say that all students hold gloriously positive opinions about alcohol. In fact, most students will readily admit that alcohol produces some problems for themselves and others. Likewise, many students acknowledge that they are sometimes disturbed by others' drinking (Wechsler et al., 1995). This may be one reason that more students are choosing to live in sober housing (Wechsler et al., 2002). In truth, most students have mixed feelings about alcohol—consistent with much of the adult population—but see it as an important part of their social world. While most young people will defend their drinking when challenged, most are equally thoughtful about their social world if given the chance to be. This means that the information students provide depends on how the question is asked. For instance, a query like "Alcohol is a terrible menace, isn't it?" will likely produce a defensive response. Students want to retain their choice to drink. A more neutral question, like "I wonder what things you have observed, both good and not-so-good, about alcohol?", typically results in a more balanced and thoughtful reply. Students, too, have mixed feelings about alcohol. For this reason, this book advocates a way of talking with college students that invites their mixed impressions about alcohol, rather than global positives or negatives.

MANAGING THE DISCONNECT

College administrators are in a sticky situation. We have described a pattern of risky alcohol use that is relatively common on American campuses, but have also noted that heavy drinking has existed for a long time, is reflected in the broader American culture, and that students, by and large, do not share administrative concerns.

While efforts to limit and curtail heavy alcohol use can be productive, they cannot be one-dimensional. Conflicted and one-sided policies lead administrators to see students as wild and rebellious and lead students to see the administration as old-fashioned and controlling. As we note in the next chapter, community health programs are most likely to succeed if they include environmental changes, institutional changes, and evidence-based interventions (Hingson & Howland, 2002). A central challenge in this process is, of course, including college students as key stakeholders.

In this book we describe a set of individual and group exercises that can effectively engage students and minimize the harms associated with alcohol. These strategies, drawn from motivational and cognitive-behavioral interventions, are intended to encourage a more productive dialogue between students and providers about alcohol use. College staff have many opportunities to talk with students about alcohol, ranging from very brief conversations to formal counseling sessions. However, because we focus primarily on change at the individual level, our suggestions must be part of a larger effort to minimize the harms of college drinking.

KEY POINTS

- Drinking, and occasional heavy drinking, is relatively common among U.S. adults and especially among young adults. About 40% of college students report drinking five or more drinks in one episode in the past 2 weeks. College students tend to drink more (but use fewer other substances) than young adults who are not enrolled in college.
- Although about 40% students drink heavily at times, consistently heavy use is reported by about 19%.
- Heavy drinking in college is most often centered on events and opportunities to drink and is likely less consistent than might be implied by survey questionnaires.
- College drinking rates have remained relatively stable over the last 20 years, but may have increased over the last 50 years. College women, in particular, drink more than they did in the 1950s.
- There is wide variation in rates of heavy drinking from one college to the next.
- Alcohol use is related to a range of difficulties, including lower GPA, higher rates of intoxicated driving and violence, and greater problems for others on campus.
- In general, students are less concerned about alcohol than are other members of the community. Most have mixed feelings about alcohol but still see drinking (and occasional heavy drinking) as part of the normal college experience.

2

Responding to College Drinking

OVERVIEW OF THE CHAPTER

In this chapter, we present the background and rationale for the recommendations we make in later chapters. We first review conceptual models of college drinking—the "why students drink?" question. We then review models of prevention and intervention—the "how do we help students?" question—and discuss how our recommendations fit in. If you are mainly interested in the clinical aspects of this book, look over the key points at the end of this chapter and skip to the next chapter. But if you are curious about *why* we recommend what we do, then read on.

Unfortunately, there does not appear to be a single or simple explanation for why students drink or why some interventions work better than others. In making recommendations, we consider research about college drinking broadly, borrow from different conceptual and treatment approaches, and recommend interventions that have support in the research literature. Most generally, we base our approach on a public health model. We also believe that the strategies of motivational interviewing (MI) and cognitive-behavioral therapy (CBT) offer good options for helping individual students reduce their drinking-related risk.

MODELS OF ALCOHOL PROBLEMS

How do alcohol problems arise? There is no shortage of models for understanding why humans consume alcohol in ways that cause problems. For a full discussion of these models, we refer readers to an excellent chapter by Miller and Hester (2003), which discusses 13 different conceptual models of alcohol use and problems, including those based on *moral* grounds, *spirituality*, *disease* processes, *genetics*, *biology*, *learning* history, *character*, and *society and culture*. Each model holds somewhat different assumptions about the nature of alcohol problems and makes somewhat different recommendations about what is helpful in prevention and treatment. For example, from a *moral* perspective, alcohol problems result from a lack of personal responsibility and self-control and can be remedied by moral suasion and social and legal sanctions. A perspective based in *biology* suggests that alcohol problems are largely due to heredity and brain physiology and can be changed through risk identification, genetic counseling, and medical treatment. A *sociocultural* model holds that alcohol problems are the result of social norms and environmental influences and can be remedied through changes in price, distribution, and other social policies. To review all the evidence for and implications of these models is beyond our scope. Suffice it to say that there is some evidence for each model, but each is also limited as a single explanation of all alcohol problems.

After reviewing the various models, Miller and Hester (2003) advocate for an approach grounded in *theories of public health*—a suggestion we enthusiastically support. From a public health perspective, three factors determine alcohol use: the *agent* (in this case, alcohol), the *host* (the person and their individual risk factors), and the *environment* (the context in which host meets agent). Each of these levels is thus a target for prevention and intervention efforts. From a public health perspective, prevention or treatment strategies based on other conceptual models can be incorporated at these different levels if they are shown to be effective.

COLLEGE STUDENTS AND RISK

What factors are related to alcohol use among college students? At a basic level, the *agent*, alcohol, is a toxin that humans enjoy in small doses but can be harmful if consumed in large-enough quantities. Small amounts of alcohol may have health benefits with respect to heart disease, particularly for middle-aged white males (Gunzerath, Faden, Zakhari, & Warren, 2004; Mukamal et al., 2003), but large amounts can damage a number of body organs, particularly the liver and brain ("Medical Consequences," 2000). As noted in Chapter 1, every year a few college students die from alcohol poisoning, but, for the most part, physiological damage is rare in those ages 18–25 ("Medical Consequences," 2000). Rather, younger people tend to suffer more from accidents and the social and legal consequences of drinking. Drinkers can also become psychologically or physically dependent on the drug effects of alcohol, although, as noted in Chapter 1, this is less common among college students than among older drinkers.

In terms of *individual*, or "*host*" factors, researchers have identified a number of potential variables, such as family history, personality, beliefs in alcohol's effects, perceived norms, stress, and anxiety. There is no one type of college drinker nor is there a simple or single reason for drinking within this age group. However, some patterns have emerged. In particular, students who are more *impulsive* and *disinhibited* consistently report more alcohol-related problems (Baer, 2002; Ham & Hope, 2003). In general, students who like to take risks, hold more positive beliefs about the effects of alcohol, or have a history of antisocial behavior drink more and have more problems than other kinds of students. This relationship—that impulsive students drink more and have and cause more problems—is perhaps the most consistent finding in the last 30 years of research on predictors of college drinking.

A second relationship—between *stress and depression* and alcohol use—is also supported in the literature (Baer, 2002; Ham & Hope, 2003). In short, depressed and anxious students are more likely to abuse alcohol and have alcohol-related problems. Sadly, these kinds of students rarely come to the attention of college officials because they do not break rules in the same rowdy manner as do their more disinhibited peers. This pattern probably constitutes a smaller share of college drinking than the impulsive pattern. However, it may be associated with alcohol problems that persist after college (Kushner, Sher, & Erickson, 1999).

A third pattern is that young people who are more *social* tend to drink more (Baer, 2002). We noted in Chapter 1 that students see alcohol as an important part of their social world. The relationship seems intuitive: College students tend to drink in social contexts, and, thus, those who are more social are more likely to drink. The irony is that sociability and extraversion are not consistently related to drinking in either older or younger populations (Wood, Vinson, & Sher, 2001). For instance, among middle-aged adults, extraversion and sociability do not consistently predict greater alcohol use—most social middle-aged persons drink moderately. Likewise, many of the most social younger adolescents drink little or not at all. The college years seem to be different in this respect, and at this point, sociability seems to be a key risk factor for heavy drinking.

In addition to variables that do predict drinking, there is one risk factor that usually does *not* predict drinking among college students. Although genetic risk factors—having blood relatives with alcohol problems—are associated with alcohol problems in the general population, they tend not to be consistently related to drinking during the college years (Baer, 2002). Two explanations appear likely. First, many adolescents with severe alcohol and drug problems do not enroll in college, and this minimizes our ability to see genetic effects within the subpopulation of young adults who are enrolled. Second, alcohol and drug problems associated with genetic differences may emerge later in life, after longer periods of use.

Aside from individual factors, *environmental* factors also influence college student health and safety. Contextual factors that predict drinking come in many shapes and sizes—some proximal, like the drinking of peers and close friends, and some more distal, like the price and availability of alcohol and the density of retail outlets near campus (Presley et al., 2002; Weitzman, Folkman, Folkman, & Wechsler, 2003). Among these environmental factors, peer use is the single best predictor of rates of individual alcohol use. There is some evidence for two different social influence processes here: socialization and selection (Sher et al., 2001). In other words, students tend to seek out friends who share their interests and activities—in this case, drinking. Students also tend to share the habits of their closest friends. In fact, estimates of friends' drinking are pretty good predictors of how much an individual drinks him- or herself (Kypri & Langley, 2003). Certain social activities, such as membership in fraternities and sororities or on athletic teams, are also associated with greater drinking and related problems (Cashin, Presley, & Meilman, 1998; Leichliter, Meilman, Presley, & Cashin, 1998). Finally, students who live on campus tend to drink more than those who commute (Valliant & Scanlan, 1996).

Do individual and environmental factors interact? For instance, is it particularly risky for an impulsive or disinhibited individual to live with others who drink a lot? We'll waffle here, but only a little. At this point, there is not much evidence for a *multiplicative* effect of personal and environmental factors. It is a reasonable assumption though, and research support may not be far off. There is little doubt that individual and environmental factors are at least *additive*. That is, risk factors seem to contribute individually, but may also sum to create ultimate risk. By this logic, we should be most concerned about a college student who has a history of problems with rules, makes decisions impulsively, is a member of a fraternity, whose close friends are heavy drinkers, and who resides at a university that has many retail outlets nearby and a culture tolerant of heavy drinking.

DRINKING AND DEVELOPMENT

We cannot end this discussion about the "whys" of college drinking without mentioning an additional, complicating factor: time. None of these three categories of risk—agent, host, or environment—exists independent of the fact that young people are growing and changing. The transition, in both physical and psychological terms, from an adolescent attending high school to a young adult at a college or university, is enormous. The college period is a time of inherent and sometimes chaotic change. Young peoples' living situations change (assuming a move from the home), as do their friendships, personal and career goals, and even self-image. This time of upheaval creates both opportunities and risks. On the one hand, young people become more competent and independent and develop a more adult view of their own preferences and abilities. On the other hand, young people may also suffer from stress and health and safety risks.

Schulenberg and Maggs (2002) have thoughtfully reviewed some of the developmental issues that affect college drinking. They note that, in theory, the many physical and psychological demands at this age can overload coping abilities, create mismatches between needs and resources, and heighten vulnerability to chance events. Attention to developmental processes has led Arnett (2000) to suggest a new developmental period for the ages of 18–25, called "emerging adulthood." He argues that individuals within this rough age span are distinct demographically and psychologically from both younger (adolescent) and older (adult) age groups. In many Western cultures, young people may stay in educational systems and delay marriage and parenthood until well into their 20s or 30s. Within emerging adulthood, identity explorations in the areas of love, work, and worldview go beyond the initial formulations made in adolescence but stop short of adulthood.

How does development relate to drinking? There are two concepts we want to emphasize. First, consistent with much of life during this period, *changing* alcohol use is the rule.

This pattern was documented by Schulenberg, O'Malley, Bachman, Wadsworth, and Johnston (1996) who used the MTF database to examine heavy drinking during the ages of 18–23. Heavy drinking over this time was reported *consistently* by only 7% of respondents. It was more much common for these young adults to report heavy drinking sporadically (17%) or at one point but not others (10%, a "fling"). It was also common for young people to report patterns of either increasing (10%) or decreasing (12%) drinking over time. Thus, the same risky behavior at any point in time (e.g., heavy episodic drinking) could be a part of any of five long-term patterns (sporadic, fling, regular, increasing, or decreasing). This means that larger drinking patterns are more complicated than the data gathered from a single drinking episode. In the MTF data, as well as in our own (Weingardt et al., 1998), students who drank heavily *and* consistently had many more negative consequences. And, of course, an increasing or chronic pattern of use would be associated with greater risks than would a decreasing or infrequent pattern of use. Finally, as noted in Chapter 1, heavy drinking more often than not remits once individuals graduate or leave college. Thus, alcohol use among college students most often, but not always, represents a *period* of risk during life.

The second way that development affects drinking is in terms of the many psychological tasks of this period. Arnett (2000) proposes that heavy drinking is a part of the *role exploration and self-exploration* that is common during this developmental period. Drinking may help establish or define a young adult's *adulthood or independence*. Likewise, Schulenberg and Maggs (2002) suggest that young adults sometimes use alcohol to *cope with stress associated with developmental transitions*. Alcohol may help a student make new friends or fit in socially. Drinking might also be a part of a young adult's attempt to act and feel independent.

In summary, rather than being a simple rebellious act, college drinking is a complex social behavior that results from important environmental and psychological influences. Students not only vary with respect to how much they drink, but with respect to *why* they drink. Unfortunately, there is no single cause of college student drinking—it is multi-determined (NIAAA, 2002). Likewise, there appears to be no single pattern that is more risky or troublesome than others; risk comes in many shapes and sizes. Research on individual factors has given us a few clues as to what factors place people more at risk (e.g., impulsivity, stress and coping, and socializing), as well as what the most important environmental influences are. We also know that risk for alcohol-related problems is at least additive. In general, the more risk factors, the more risk. As emerging adults, college students are trying on adult behaviors, exploring new roles and self-images, and managing a time of great transition in terms of personal goals, relationships, and activities.

WHEN CHANGE OCCURS

When it comes to college drinking, change is more common than stability. This raises the obvious question: What makes students change their drinking? Although there is much we don't know about how and why people change, we have a few clues. First, we know that most people make changes without formal assistance, even those with severe drinking problems (Finney, Moos, & Timko, 1999; Sobell, Cunningham, & Sobell, 1996). At a philosophical level, we also assume that college students are autonomous individuals who make choices about their personal and social behavior. Students choose to drink because, given the contingencies of time and place, they want to. In the same way, students can also choose to drink less, when the risks of use outweigh the perceived benefits or when the benefits of drinking *moderately* outweigh the benefits of drinking *a lot*. For instance, a student might curtail his or her drinking when he or she wants to avoid a hangover or embarrassment, perceives drunkenness as outside the norm, needs to do well on an exam or for a job, no longer sees alcohol as a way to separate from parents or fit in socially, or when alcohol is too expensive or difficult to obtain.

Like all changes, changes in drinking do not usually occur all at once. Our work with college students is generally informed by the transtheoretical model of behavior change (TTM; Prochaska, DiClemente, & Norcross, 1992). This now well-known model proposes that change happens in more-or-less discrete stages: (1) *precontemplation*, in which a person has no interest in or intent to change; (2) *contemplation*, in which a person is aware that a change might be beneficial and is considering taking action; (3) *preparation*, in which an individual is intending to take action soon; (4) *action*, in which a person is actively modifying his or her behavior or environment; and (5) *maintenance*, in which a person is working to maintain changes he or she has already made and to avoid relapse to old behaviors. Figure 2.1 illustrates the different stages. Based on studies of how people change addictive and other health behaviors, researchers have identified certain cognitive processes that people commonly use to navigate each of the stages. For instance, cognitive or affective processes, such as consciousness raising and environmental reevaluation, are used more

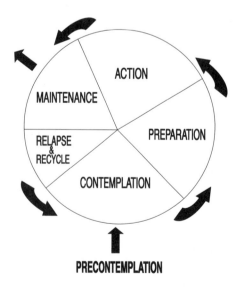

FIGURE 2.1. Transtheoretical stages of change. From Velasquez, Maurer, Crouch, and DiClemente (2001). Copyright 2001 by The Guilford Press. Reprinted by permission.

frequently in the precontemplation stage; commitment consolidation processes, such as self-reevaluation, are more frequent during the contemplation and preparation stages; and behavioral or coping strategies are more frequent during the preparation and action stages (DiClemente et al., 1991; Prochaska et al., 1992).

In working with college students, we have found the stages-of-change model extremely helpful. It suggests that change is a natural and dynamic process, as individuals reexamine their choices in light of experience. From it, we can also extrapolate two important suggestions for those who work with college students. First, the TTM suggests that effective prevention and treatment approaches *facilitate movement along the stages of change*. If a precontemplative student becomes contemplative, he or she has taken a step in the right direction. This makes our intervention goal more attainable. Our immediate goal need not always be a behavioral endpoint (e.g., safe drinking or abstinence), but might be a positive shift in thinking about change. That is, effective programs need not result in immediate reductions or cessation of alcohol use. Raising the awareness of a precontemplative student can be a success in and of itself.

Second, the TTM suggests ways to develop stage-specific interventions, through *targeting the specific psychological processes associated with movement from one stage to another*. In other words, certain facts and information should be emphasized, depending on the stage. For instance, a person in the action stage benefits most from strategies that support efforts to change, such as concrete plans. In contrast, an individual in the precontemplation stage, which in our opinion represents the majority of college students, benefits most from consciousness-raising strategies (e.g., highlighting personal drinking patterns, related consequences, alcohol expectancies) and environmental reevaluation (e.g., highlighting campus drinking norms). Precontemplators may hold misperceptions about alcohol, believing that heavy alcohol use is more common and accepted than it actually is or that alcohol produces significant positive effects. A reexamination of these beliefs about alcohol's effects and about social norms with respect to use thus becomes the focus of prevention programming for students in the precontemplation and contemplation stages. Indeed, research has shown that tailoring an intervention to an individual's stage of change generally increases its effectiveness (Perz, DiClemente, & Carbonari, 1996).[1]

IMPLICATIONS FOR INTERVENTION

This understanding of young adults, alcohol, and change points us away from some prevention and intervention approaches and toward others. Programs that address only one risk factor will probably have limited impact. For instance, an intervention that targets the problematic drinking resulting from stress and depression would obviously not work well for the more common social or disinhibited drinkers. Systems designed to find and treat alcoholic students would similarly miss the vast majority of individuals. And, of course, an

---

[1]For a more detailed discussion of ways to integrate this model into treatment, including specific techniques that are most useful at different stages, see Connors, Donovan, and DiClemente (2001).

intervention based on faulty assumptions would be ineffective altogether. For example, a program designed to identify and warn those most at risk for genetic problems (e.g., children of alcoholic parents) would probably not affect most college drinkers. Educational or counseling services that simply tell students what they are "supposed" to do will run headlong into developmental processes of identity development. Finally, any effort that assumes most students already want to change will miss the majority who have not yet seriously considered the possibility.

In contrast to approaches based on a single risk factor, prevention and intervention programs targeted to precontemplative or contemplative emerging adults who may have a range of risk factors are likely to be beneficial to many more students. These include efforts to raise awareness of the negative consequences of heavy drinking and those that seek to highlight the benefits of abstinence or careful moderate drinking. Approaches that address misperceptions about alcohol effects or drinking norms should likewise bring choices into sharper relief. Best of all, programs that seek to reduce alcohol use while simultaneously supporting autonomy and other developmental processes should be more acceptable to students and, therefore, more effective.

WHAT WORKS IN PREVENTION AND TREATMENT?

Given the discussion above, how do we prevent or minimize harms associated with college drinking? What can we recommend? We are once again fortunate to have several recent literature reviews to draw from. The most comprehensive is the recent National Institute on Alcohol Abuse and Alcoholism (NIAAA) Task Force Report on college drinking (NIAAA, 2002),[2] which in many ways is a review of reviews (Larimer & Cronce, 2002; DeJong & Langford, 2002; Perkins, 2002; Walters & Bennett, 2000). The task force, consisting of college presidents, academic researchers, and student representatives, was charged to review the causes of collegiate drinking and make recommendations for addressing the problem. The resulting report is organized into tiers that reflect the quantity and quality of empirical support for different kinds of approaches.

At the time of the report, there was surprisingly little research to draw from. Despite the many anecdotal accounts of success, most programs have not been tested using good research designs. Moreover, among those programs that have research support, outcome measures have often been used that would be considered substandard in other areas of evaluative research, such as qualitative measures (e.g., satisfaction with the program), prospective estimates of change (e.g., how much the student thinks he or she will change as a result), or changes in something other than drinking (e.g., knowledge of alcohol-related facts). Surprisingly, most outcome studies don't measure changes in drinking. In addition, college campuses differ in many student and institutional variables, making it difficult to know if interventions that are successful on one campus will generalize to others.

---

[2]The final report is available at www.collegedrinkingprevention.gov.

Limitations aside, the task force did make some clear recommendations for colleges seeking to implement effective programs. In their first tier, the task force listed approaches showing *clear evidence of effectiveness*—those programs tested with strong research designs and that resulted in encouraging outcomes. In particular, there was good evidence that cognitive-behavioral skills training and motivational counseling approaches could reduce drinking. In addition, briefer programs that employed motivational strategies and alcohol expectancy challenges were also effective. Program duration did not predict outcome; shorter programs were, on average, as effective as longer programs. Most of these first-tier programs had been tested as *indicated prevention*, that is, with students who were already heavy drinkers. In addition, most had been evaluated with volunteer subjects, typically screened out of psychology testing pools. Very few had been done "in the field" with nonvolunteer high-risk students. Nevertheless, it is noteworthy that most of these programs involved individual or group interactions between staff and students.

The task force included a second tier consisting mostly of *universal prevention* approaches that showed *good evidence of effectiveness in other populations but had not been specifically tested with college students*. These approaches included increased enforcement of minimum-age drinking laws, restrictions on alcohol retail outlet density, better implementation and enforcement of laws related to drinking and driving, increased price of alcohol, responsible beverage-service policies, and the formation of campus and community coalitions to support policy implementation.

Finally, a number of additional universal prevention programs were included in a third tier, where evidence was lacking but where the committee felt there was a promising theoretical rationale. These approaches included the establishment of alcohol-free residences for students, banning alcohol at alumni and faculty events, increased enforcement of alcohol policies at campus events, and social norms marketing campaigns.

The task force also made a clear statement that, though theoretically reasonable, some programs have been tested and found *ineffective*. In a fourth tier, the task force noted that there was good evidence that informational, knowledge-based, and values clarification programs, when used alone, were typically *not effective* in changing alcohol use. Nor was the provision of blood alcohol level feedback, again when used in isolation, effective. Table 2.1 summarizes the resulting framework for addressing alcohol use at the individual, campus, and community level.

HOW THIS BOOK FITS IN

We agree with the NIAAA Task Force and other writers that there is a culture of heavy drinking on most college campuses. Changes to this culture will ultimately require broad-based, integrated community responses. *This book focuses on one aspect of the community response—individual and group interactions.* Although the problem of heavy drinking in college cannot be fixed solely through face-to-face interactions, we believe that the approaches we outline in this book are an important part of the mix and likely to be helpful

TABLE 2.1. Three-in-One Framework for Campus Alcohol Prevention

Tier	Strategy
1. Effective among college students	• Combining cognitive-behavioral skills with norms clarification and motivational enhancement interventions • Offering brief motivational enhancement interventions in student health centers and emergency rooms • Challenging alcohol expectancies
2. Effective with general populations	• Increased enforcement of minimum drinking age laws • Implementation, increased publicity, and enforcement of other laws to reduce alcohol-impaired driving • Restrictions on alcohol retail density • Increased price and excise taxes on alcoholic beverages • Responsible beverage service policies in social and commercial settings • The formation of a campus–community coalition
3. Promising	• Adopting campus-based policies to reduce high-risk use (e.g., reinstating Friday classes, eliminating keg parties, establishing alcohol-free activities and dorms) • Increasing enforcement at campus-based events that promote excessive drinking • Increasing publicity about enforcement of underage drinking laws/eliminating "mixed" messages • Consistently enforcing campus disciplinary actions associated with policy violations • Conducting marketing campaigns to correct student misperception about alcohol use on campus • Provision of "safe rides" programs • Regulation of happy hours and sales • Enhancing awareness of personal liability • Informing new students and parents about alcohol policies and penalties
4. Ineffective	• Informational, knowledge-based, or values clarification interventions when used alone

Note. From National Institute on Alcohol Abuse and Alcoholism (2002).

to many students (see Chapter 8 for a discussion of service integration). Talking with students in ways that are effective *can* reduce drinking and related harm. Counseling and other face-to-face interactions can also reinforce messages from media and public health campaigns. As we develop more fully in the next chapter, counseling can serve the function of assessment and referral as well, linking students with services that are more tailored to their needs.

In the chapters that follow, we present a series of techniques and strategies that are used to interact face-to-face with college students about alcohol. We believe that these strategies reflect those with the greatest empirical support as reviewed by the NIAAA Task

Force. The strategies draw on a number of motivational assumptions—in particular that students can and do weigh the pros and cons of their behavior, that there are strong influences to drink and good reasons to be careful if choosing to drink, and that students should become more contemplative about their choices. *If we approach students with a clear message, using a style that does not make them defensive, we can facilitate change.* We also believe that college students are growing, changing, and developing. Alcohol use, and especially heavy use, during this time is best thought of as a developmental period or *window of risk*—one that is most often time-limited and that we wish to minimize in length and intensity.

Last, and perhaps most important, techniques like those presented in this book need not be employed solely by therapists in counseling centers. For this reason, we use the terms *counseling* and *counselor* loosely. In practice, students interact with concerned others in a wide array of settings—from formal interventions in counseling centers to educational programs delivered by prevention staff, brief advice from staff at health centers, informal conferences with parents and concerned others, and frequent small conversations with faculty or residence hall staff. All these encounters are opportunities to encourage contemplation of the risks of drinking. Because we want to engage students during these interactions, the material in the subsequent chapters is a toolbox of strategies that can be used to change the conversation with college students. Many of these strategies can be brief, opportunistic, and delivered by nonspecialists. In this way, effective individual and group interactions can be used to reach a larger number of students and ultimately affect the campus culture.

ORGANIZING THE TOOLBOX

Opportunities for talking with students about alcohol come in many shapes and sizes. However, we recognize that most college service providers have real constraints on the way they can interact with students. For this reason, we organize our suggestions based on available time. Following distinctions suggested by Rollnick and colleagues (2002), we suggest two brief models and one longer one. Very brief encounters (e.g., 5–10 minutes)— what we call *brief advice*—are based on medical consultation research (Dunn, 2003; Emmen, Schippers, Bleijenberg, & Wollersheim, 2004; Rollnick, Mason, & Butler, 1999). There is some evidence from research in healthcare settings that these ultra-brief encounters can be effective at reducing drinking. For slightly longer encounters (e.g., 10–30 minutes), we recommend what we call *behavioral consultation*. Compared to brief advice, there are fewer tests of this model, but the techniques have a solid theoretical base. Behavioral consultation expands on brief advice through the use of a few simple motivational techniques. If you have more individual time with a student, we recommend the more structured assessment and counseling protocol described in Chapter 6, a *motivational intervention*. This model has strong support in the literature (Burke, Arkowitz, & Dunn, 2002; Larimer & Cronce, 2001; Walters & Bennett, 2000) and would be our choice as the "gold standard" intervention for heavy-drinking students. If you have more than 50 minutes or have multiple interactions with a student, we suggest other motivational activities that might be helpful. In Chapter 7, we describe the use of MI principles with groups of students. There is less research on motivational groups, but we can make some suggestions based on the research literature and our clinical experience conducting these groups. Although we have tried to assemble coherent, self-contained interactions, providers should feel free to add or subtract elements as is appropriate to particular goals and context. Finally, in Chapter 8, we make suggestions for how these models might be integrated into broader, community-level programs.

KEY POINTS

- A number of factors influence the way college students drink. A public health model looks at the problem broadly, taking into account *agent*, *host*, and *environmental* factors.
- In general, college students are more likely to drink if they are male, white, or belong to fraternities, sororities, or athletic teams. Students who are more impulsive, depressed, or social also tend to drink more and have more related problems. Genetic factors are not strongly related to drinking during college. Access to alcohol and permissive campus norms are associated with greater drinking problems.
- As students grow, drinking patterns tend to change. Most students reduce their risky use once they leave college.
- Most college students are, at best, contemplative about their drinking and do not see it as a problem. When change occurs, it most often happens naturally, without formal treatment services.
- Individual programs are most effective when they are tailored to an individual student's stage of change. Raising awareness of the dangers of risky alcohol use or the benefits of moderate drinking or abstinence is a valuable goal in and of itself.
- In general, programs that use motivational and cognitive-behavioral strategies and programs that target policy changes are most effective at reducing drinking.
- An integrated community response is required to change the culture of heavy drinking on college campuses.

3

Assessing Drinking and Related Behaviors

OVERVIEW OF THE CHAPTER

Assessment is the first step in programs tailored to the individual.[1] We noted in Chapter 1 that there is considerable drinking variability among college students. In this chapter, we suggest ways to evaluate an individual's drinking and related issues and make decisions based on this information. There are several reasons it is important to understand an individual student's drinking:

- Information about drinking allows us to refer or match students to appropriate services. We want to know *what*, *why*, and *how* a student drinks so that we can direct him or her to services that are most likely to be helpful.
- Information about drinking allows us to tailor what we or someone else says or does. Information about alcohol use and consequences, as well as attitudes and beliefs, can be used as the content or focus of prevention or treatment programs.
- Sincere and candid questions let a student know that we are interested in him or her. If conducted with good interviewing skills, questions can also communicate concern and empathy. They allow us to speak directly to the individual's experiences.

Assessment is not difficult, but getting ready to assess can be. It requires that we select certain questions from myriad options. This chapter presents options for assessment and, where possible, notes benefits and limitations of the different approaches. The context of the interaction—how we come into contact with students and how much time we have—will naturally affect options and choices. A 5-minute assessment in a student health center will look different from a 2-hour assessment in a psychology clinic, even though their purposes might overlap. In this chapter, we briefly review some of places where

---

[1]A prevention program targeted to an entire population typically would not include individual assessment.

assessment is used and make suggestions for best practices given different goals and settings. In Chapters 5 and 6, we provide additional suggestions for when and where different assessments might make sense when paired with different interventions. Finally, in Appendices A–E, we provide copies of several measures we have found especially helpful. Those who have only very brief interactions with students might want to concentrate on the Alcohol Consumption (p. 27) and Alcohol Screening (p. 35) sections of this chapter, which suggest ways to assess briefly how much a student is drinking and to determine whether to refer him or her for more specialized services.

This chapter is not intended as a complete review of drinking assessment, especially assessment related to research and program evaluation. Assessment for these purposes is explored in a large and complex literature; fortunately, the NIAAA (2004) has produced an excellent volume, *Assessing Alcohol Problems*, that discusses and reproduces many of the tests. In this chapter, we choose measures selectively based on their clinical use with college students. Research on college assessments is unfortunately limited, so in many cases we have had to take our best guess in making recommendations.

Our discussion is divided into three sections. We begin by reviewing assessments of *alcohol involvement*, including drinking rate, drinking-related negative consequences, and alcohol dependence. Next, we review *screening measures* that tap aspects of these dimensions. We finish by briefly noting options for *related areas*—problem recognition, beliefs in alcohol effects, drinking contexts, and family history of alcohol problems. In each section we give our preferences, and at the end of the chapter we provide a table that summarizes our recommendations.

A final note before we begin: Nearly all college alcohol assessments are self-report. In the past, individual self-reports about drinking have often been assumed to be biased. This is perhaps due to the historical notions that alcoholics are in denial and chronically lie to conceal their condition or that people won't admit to embarrassing things. However, considerable research suggests that self-reports can be reliable and valid indicators of drinking if the individual believes that he or she has nothing to lose based on the report, is sober when reporting, and is given assurances of confidentiality (Babor, Brown, & Del Boca, 1990; Maisto & Connors, 1990; Sobell & Sobell, 2004). In fact, in comparing self-reports to the reports of others, we find that college students are as likely to overestimate (brag) as they are to underestimate (minimize) their drinking (e.g., Marlatt et al., 1998). The greater problems, described below, are that students may not pay enough attention to what they are drinking or that the assessments themselves may be so vaguely worded that students have difficulty answering them accurately.

WHEN AND WHERE TO ASSESS DRINKING

University staff can use assessments in a variety of interactions. Formal appointments occur in medical, counseling, administrative, and academic settings. Sometimes appointments are brief—5 to 10 minutes for consultation on a particular topic. Informally, students also interact with faculty before and after class, talk with resident advisors in the halls, and seek information from administrative staff. Sometimes appointments are more extended, as can be the case with voluntary counseling or referrals for violations of university policy. Alcohol assessments can also be used as part of routine or specialized screenings, such as check-ins at health center visits, new student orientations, or health and wellness classes. Of course, in many of these contexts, alcohol use may have nothing to do with the reason for the appointment. In fact, our experience suggests that, more often than not, alcohol is *not* the initial or stated purpose of the meeting, even when it ultimately becomes a topic of conversation.

Obviously, the nature of assessment will vary depending on the available time and purpose of the contact. Even in a very brief encounter, one or two questions about alcohol may be appropriate. With more time, an interview can provide information about other practices and risks. In Chapter 2, we described a rough grouping of different interactions based on available time, and in Chapters 5 and 6, we present specific exercises that can be used for brief advice, behavioral consultation, and longer motivational interventions. For purposes of our discussion of assessment, we use a parallel three-level system also based on available time: brief assessment (less than 5 minutes), moderate-length assessment (5–15 minutes), and extended-length assessment (more than 15 minutes). Brief assessments are appropriate during informal meetings and discussions when one only has time to ask a few questions and the use of questionnaires might be awkward. In fact, the information gained in such a short period is necessarily quite limited and typically can only be used to support brief advice (see Chapter 5). Moderate-length assessments may allow for the use of a brief structured interview or questionnaire, in addition to other informal questions. With more than about 15 minutes for assessment, there are many more options for gathering a variety of drinking-related information.

ALCOHOL CONSUMPTION

When considering alcohol *consumption*, three dimensions are typically assessed: drinking rate or pattern, drinking-related negative consequences, and alcohol abuse or dependence diagnoses.

Drinking Rate

As noted in Chapter 1, drinking rate can be looked at in terms of frequency (i.e., how often), quantity (i.e., how much), and specific episodes of heavy drinking. Although this seems like a simple procedure, it can be much more complicated in practice. For example, at a meeting in April 2000, researchers from 12 countries met to develop standards for assessing alcohol consumption. What resulted were 12 different academic papers and a summary paper that detailed 34 recommendations (Dawson & Room, 2000). For our discussion of drinking rate, we use a simple grouping of methods suggested by Sobell and

Sobell (2004): (1) *quantity–frequency (QF)* methods, which ask the individual to give an estimate of average quantity, frequency, or peak consumption over a period of time; and (2) *daily drinking (DD)* methods, which ask the individual to estimate how much he or she drank each day during an interval.

QF methods are commonly used in survey research. As described in Chapter 1, college students might be asked a question like:

> *How frequently have you consumed alcoholic beverages (beer, wine, spirits) over the past 90 days?*
> _____ *Not at all*
> _____ *Less than once a month*
> _____ *One to two times a month*
> _____ *One to two times a week*
> _____ *Three to four times a week*
> _____ *Daily or almost daily*

A student's answer gives an estimate of the total number of times he or she consumed alcohol in a typical day, week, or month during this 90-day window. Of course, in a more informal setting, the student could be asked the same question without the categories.

Drinking *quantity* is slightly more complicated. As we mentioned in Chapter 1, different types of alcohol are made comparable by defining a "standard drink," typically described as 12 ounces of beer, 4 ounces of wine, or 1¼ ounces of 80-proof spirits. For instance:

> *When consuming beverages containing alcohol, on average, how many drinks do you have in one sitting? (A "drink" is defined as 12 ounces of beer, 4 ounces of wine, or 1¼ ounces of 80-proof spirits):*
> _____ *One drink*
> _____ *Two to three drinks*
> _____ *Four to five drinks*
> _____ *Six to seven drinks*
> _____ *Seven to eight drinks*
> _____ *More than 8 drinks*

Again, this question can be asked in an open-ended format, without the categories. Note that the drinking categories and threshold for the highest category (e.g., "more than eight drinks") are essentially arbitrary. Some surveys use different categories that extend well into the teens.

Despite the attempt to standardize amounts, there are still many limitations to quantity measures like these. First, since beverages vary in size and alcohol content, most students are only vaguely aware of how much they are consuming or how much alcohol is in the drink. This may be particularly true at parties where students consume alcohol without knowing exactly what is in the drink (e.g., "jungle punch"). Second, keg and tap beer is usually served in cups that are bigger than the 10- to 12-ounce standard drink size, which means that students may underreport drinking. Third, despite the assumption that mixed drinks contain a consistent one shot of 80-proof liquor, restaurants routinely serve drinks that contain much more or less alcohol than this. Likewise, those who self-mix might add well beyond one shot per drink. Even within a single establishment, alcohol content can vary with time of day. For instance, an inexpensive happy hour drink may be much weaker than the same drink at other times of the day. Finally, most college students (and other adults) simply don't count how many drinks they are having. To address some of these difficulties, assessments sometimes ask separate questions for each beverage type (e.g., how many beers, how many glasses of wine, how many shots/mixed drinks?). It can also be helpful to have pictures or examples of different sizes of glasses, pitchers, and bottles to help students more accurately estimate the amount they consumed. Pitchers of beer in the United States, for example, may hold 48 or 60 ounces.

More formal research-based QF measures sometimes assess quantity and frequency of different beverage types separately (Cahalan, Cisin, & Crossley, 1969) to compute a "volume–variability" index that puts drinkers into categories. These categories can be used to identify people who tend to bunch their drinks together. Complicated QF indices lose their simplicity, however. A common alternative used in studies of college students is to define a heavy-drinking episode, and then assess its frequency. For example, in the CAS surveys, students are asked:

- [For men] *How many times have you consumed five or more drinks in a row over the last 2 weeks?*
- [For women] *How many times have you consumed four or more drinks in a row over the last 2 weeks?*

The Daily Drinking Questionnaire (DDQ) is another attempt to measure episodic drinking in a QF format (Collins, Parks, & Marlatt, 1985; Dimeff, Baer, Kivlahan, & Marlott, 1999). In this measure, students are given a weeklong calendar and are asked to write in the number of drinks typically consumed on each day. The assessment portion of the Check-Up to Go (CHUG, Appendix G) uses a similar format, with spaces on each day for different types of beverages—beer, wine, and liquor. The advantage of this format is that it allows students to differentiate between moderate drinking on some days and heavy episodes on others, although, of course, they are still averaging to create a "regular" week that may not exist. As we mentioned in Chapter 1, students tend to be opportunistic drinkers, drinking around events rather than days of the week. To account for this partially, some measures provide a separate space to describe a particularly heavy episode during the past month.

The advantage of QF measures is their brevity and simplicity. Unfortunately, QF measures don't do as good a job measuring sporadic heavy drinking, which can be especially risky. QF measures also ask for mathematical averages, which most people are not very good at estimating. As a result, QF measures tend to give lower estimates of drinking than do other kinds of measures (Sobell & Sobell, 1992).

The alternative, *daily drinking (DD) measures*, are more accurate than QF measures. DD measures, such as the Time Line Follow-Back (TLFB; Sobell, Toneatto, & Sobell, 1994) and the Form 90 (Tonigan, Miller, & Brown, 1997), use a calendar for specific period of time (e.g., the previous 90 days). Using "anchor" events, such as holidays, birthdays, and social events, individuals are asked to report how many and what kinds of alcoholic beverages they consumed on each day. Although at first blush this seems like an overwhelming task, the process actually works pretty well. Abstinent days are noted first, then regular patterns, and finally, specific instances of heavy drinking. The time it takes to complete a DD assessment varies with the length of the window (e.g., 30, 60, 90 days) and the amount of drinking the individual reports. From this assessment, any number of summary measures can be derived—frequency of drinking, average quantity, average quantity on weekends, heaviest day, etc. But the chief benefit of the DD format is the ability to capture drinking patterns without summarizing.

On the whole, DD measures generate more accurate information than do QF measures. In addition, DD methods minimize averaging and are thus more likely to reveal extreme or dangerous incidents. On the other hand, DD methods take more time to administer and require an interviewer trained in the method. These technical requirements cause most people to shy away from DD techniques, which is unfortunate. It takes time to gather accurate information about drinking.

Estimating Blood Alcohol Concentration

The most important factor in determining risk is blood alcohol concentration (BAC). This is partially because blood alcohol levels take into account the individual's gender, weight, and drinking rate.[2] Intuitively we know that five or more drinks in a row might be dangerous for a 100-pound female who drinks them all at once, but would mean little for a 200-pound male who drinks them over the course of a day. Thus, when used to make clinical decisions, assessments of drinking quantity should be adjusted based on weight, gender, and time. In Appendix J we include summary BAC cards that can help a student to estimate his or her own BAC. For a more personalized card, BAC Zone sells laminated cards that are customized based on gender and weight.[3]

To estimate peak BAC, we need gender, weight, and drinking rate. Gender and weight are usually straightforward. Those sensitive about their weight can be told that it will be helpful in calculating the amount of alcohol in their body. We also recommend asking students how long they spent drinking during a specific drinking episode. For instance, to inquire about drinking on a given evening, ask:

---

[2]BAC can also vary with food intake and hormonal fluctuations, but these differences are relatively small compared to the three main factors of gender, weight, and rate of consumption.
[3]For ordering information, see www.baczone.biz.

- *About what time did you begin drinking?*
- *About what time did you stop drinking?*

The difference between the answers is the length of the drinking episode. To calculate BAC, use the cards in Appendix J. Subtract 0.016 for each hour of drinking to arrive at the estimated peak BAC for the episode. DD techniques work well for collecting this type of information.

Some paper assessments collect information that can be used to calculate BAC. For example, the CHUG assessment (Appendix G; see also the DDQ used in Dimeff et al., 1999) asks students to write in the number of drinks they consumed on each day for different types of beverages, as well as the number of hours they spent drinking. The CHUG scoring sheet lists give websites that can automatically calculate BAC given this information. The CHUG feedback (Appendix G) also lists common experiences at different BAC levels.

Recommendations for Assessing Drinking Rate

Based on this quick review of assessment options for drinking rate, we offer the following general recommendations.

- *Be specific.* Avoid vague or closed-ended questions like "Do you drink?" and "Do you drink a lot?" Far better to ask "How many drinks did you have last Saturday night?" or "How typical was last Saturday of your drinking in the past 3 months?"
- *Limit averaging and estimating.* "How much did you drink last Saturday?" is better than "How much do you typically drink?" Similarly, "How many times have you had alcohol in the past 2 weeks?" is better than "On average, how frequently do you drink?" If using QF questions that require averaging, make intervals small (e.g., past week, past month). Assess separately by beverage type if possible.
- *Assess gender, weight, and the number of hours spent drinking during a heavy episode.* Keep this information in mind when calculating BAC.

In terms of the available time for assessment, we recommend:

- For *brief* encounters, ask two QF questions and one that taps episodic heavy drinking.
  1. *About how many times per week do you have something to drink?*
  2. *When you drink, about how many drinks do you consume in a typical day?*
  3. *During the last month, what's the most you consumed on one occasion?*
- For *moderate*-length encounters, use as much DD information as possible. Ask the student to describe a typical drinking week and one heaviest episode over the past month.

1. *If you think over the last month, how many drinks did you usually consume on a typical Monday? typical Tuesday? typical Wednesday?, etc.*
2. *During the last month, what's the most you consumed on one occasion?*
3. *On that day, when did you start drinking? When did you stop?*

- In *extended* meetings, use a DD assessment, such as the TLFB or Form 90 (see Sobell et al., 1994, or Tonigan et al., 1997, for instructions).

Negative Consequences

So much attention is given to *rates* of drinking that the *results* of drinking are often overlooked. This is unfortunate because, as we have mentioned, the consequences of drinking directly capture the things we are most interested in. Alcohol-related consequences also speak directly to the experiences of students. Students may vehemently defend their right to drink but are less likely to argue with the consequences. In addition, as we discuss in Chapters 5, 6, and 7, by highlighting the consequences of an individual's drinking, we hope to raise awareness and (if appropriate) increase the likelihood of change.

Several scales have been developed to assess drinking-related negative consequences among young adults. Among them are the Young Adult Alcohol Problems Screening Test (YAAPST; Hurlbut & Sher, 1992; Kahler, Strong, Read, Palfai, & Wood, 2004), the College Alcohol Problems Scale (CAPS and CAPS-r; Maddock, Laforge, Rossi, & O'Hare, 2001; O'Hare, 1997a), and the Drinking Practices Questionnaire (DPQ; Williams & Morrice, 1992). In addition, one scale developed for use with adolescents has been widely used with college students: the Rutgers Alcohol Problem Index (RAPI; White & Labouvie, 1989).

These scales generally ask individuals what experiences have occurred as a result of drinking and to rate the frequency of those experiences over a period of time. Items may tap obvious problems related to drinking, such as blackouts and tolerance, but might also query other experiences common to college students. For example, the YAAPST asks students, "Have you driven a car when you knew you had too much to drink to drive safely?" "Have you ever gotten into trouble at work or school because of drinking?" and "Have you ever received a lower grade on an exam or paper than you should have because of your drinking?"

There are several good consequence measures that can be completed in 5–10 minutes. The YAAPST contains 27 items (although Kahler et al., 2004, suggest that a 20-item version is just as informative), while the RAPI contains 23 items. The CAPS-r (Maddock et al., 2001) is even briefer—only 8 items—and is designed to tap two dimensions of alcohol problems: social (i.e., sexuality and driving) and personal (i.e., depression, sleep, irritability). Bear in mind that the purpose of these questions is to identify problems, not to diagnose dependence. As such, they do not generally have "cut" scores that will identify students at special risk. Also, most drinkers will report some negative consequences, so the endorsement of a few items should not be alarming in and of itself. Rather, these tests are useful for understanding students' individual experiences with alcohol. They show the interviewer *how* and *how often* alcohol has interfered with a student's life. Such information can also be included in personalized feedback, a motivational tool discussed in Chapter 5.

Recommendations for Assessing Consequences

In brief encounters, questionnaires may take too much time. For a brief assessment of consequences, we suggest asking a few questions about the student's personal experiences that are most relevant to the goals of the conversation. For example, a worker in a student health center might choose questions about physical risks:

1. *How often in the past month have you driven a car shortly after drinking three or more drinks?*
2. *How often in the past month have you had a physical injury when you were drinking?*

In an academic counseling center, you might select experiences associated with academic performance:

1. *How often in the past month have you missed class because of drinking?*
2. *How often in the past month have you performed poorly on a test because of drinking?*

For moderate-length interactions, use the eight-item CAPS-r (see Appendix C). For extended interactions, use the YAAPST (see Appendix B).

Alcohol Dependence

We recommend assessing alcohol abuse and dependence only when there is time to explore symptoms carefully and when such information is clearly warranted. An assessment of alcohol dependence makes sense when students have repeatedly come to the attention of administrators, when previous interventions have been unsuccessful, or when placement in more intensive programs requires a diagnosis. The assessment of dependence symptoms can also be useful in other applications. For example, in providing personalized feedback, some students are shocked to learn that they already meet two criteria for alcohol dependence, even though they have only been drinking for a short period of time. In addition, group discussions of the nature of dependence can sometimes be informative and motivating.

As we discussed in Chapter 1, alcohol dependence is less common among college students than among older drinkers. As such, a diagnosis is usually not necessary to gain access to most college counseling programs. Furthermore, a diagnosis of alcohol dependence can take as long as 30–45 minutes. Table 3.1 summarizes the DSM-IV criteria for

TABLE 3.1. DSM–IV Substance Dependence Criteria

Tolerance
   Needs increased amounts of alcohol to achieve the same effect, or has a reduced effect given the same amount of alcohol.
Withdrawal
   Either a physical withdrawal when alcohol is removed, or alcohol (or a closely related substance) is used to avoid withdrawal.
Impaired control
   Persistent desire or unsuccessful attempts to cut down or control drinking.
Increased consumption
   Drinking in larger amounts or over a longer period than intended.
Neglect of activities
   Important social, occupational, or recreational activities are given up or reduced because of drinking.
Time spent drinking
   A great deal of time is spent obtaining alcohol, using it, or recovering from its effects.
Use despite problems
   Continued use despite knowledge of physical or psychological problems caused or exacerbated by alcohol.

---

alcohol dependence. To receive a formal diagnosis of alcohol dependence, an individual must meet three of these criteria during a 12-month period and their presence must cause "clinically significant impairment or distress" (American Psychiatric Association, 1994).

For alcohol abuse, a less severe diagnosis, only one of the following criteria must be met during a 12-month period, and its presence must again cause "clinically significant impairment or distress":

- Failure to fulfill major role obligations
- Use in hazardous situations
- Legal problems
- Use despite interpersonal problems

Recommendations for Assessing Alcohol Dependence

Alcohol dependence can only be assessed in extended meetings. We recommend a standardized interview based on DSM-IV criteria, such as a checklist (see Hudziak et al., 1993 for a DSM-III-R version), the Structured Clinical Interview for DSM-IV (First, Spitzer, Gibbon, & Williams, 1995), or the Composite International Diagnostic Interview (Robins et al., 1989). Each of these interviews systematically queries abuse and dependence criteria, using specifically worded questions. Though comprehensive, there are also a number of trade-offs to using structured interviews, and the interested reader is referred to Maisto, McKay, and Tiffany (2004) for a thorough discussion. In most college treatment contexts, we prefer brevity. A checklist modified for DSM-IV from earlier versions (Hudziak et al.,

1993; see also Forman, Svikis, Montoya, & Blaine, 2004) takes the least amount of time and is preferred for that reason.

The Alcohol Dependence Scale (Skinner & Horn, 1984) offers a questionnaire-based option to the clinical interview. This 25-item questionnaire covers a range of cognitive, physiological, and behavioral aspects of alcohol dependence. Although not specially based on DSM criteria, the scale has good validity when compared against diagnostic interviews. A score of 9 or higher suggests high probability of some alcohol dependence (Ross, Gavin, & Skinner, 1990).

ALCOHOL SCREENING

In recent years, there has been considerable interest in developing brief and reliable measures to screen for *potential* alcohol-related problems. Alcohol screening measures are often used in primary care settings, where large groups of people present with health concerns. In our opinion, if campus medical practitioners regularly screened students in this way, the number of problem drinkers who slip through the cracks would be greatly reduced. Alcohol screening may also be appropriate in campus health centers, health classes, and other administrative and counseling offices.

Screening questionnaires come in various lengths—from as little as 3 questions to as many as 30 (see Connors & Volk, 2004, for a review). One simple screen for alcohol problems is the CAGE (Ewing, 1984; Mayfield, McLeod, & Hall, 1974), an acronym for four questions related to the desire to *C*ut down, feeling *A*nnoyed by criticism, feeling *G*uilty about drinking, and needing alcohol in the morning (*E*ye-opener). Given how nonspecific and extreme these items are, it is surprising that the CAGE works at all. But surprisingly, this simple measure is often quite effective in detecting severe alcohol problems in some populations (see Kitchens, 1994, for a review). Unfortunately, the CAGE does a poor job identifying alcohol problems among younger or less severe drinkers (Heck & Lichtenberg, 1990; Smith, Collins, Kreisberg, Volpicelli, & Alterman, 1987). This is also true of another popular screening tool, the Michigan Alcoholism Screening Test (MAST; Selzer, 1971) and the Brief MAST (Pokorny, Miller, & Kaplan, 1972; see Clements, 1998, for a thoughtful review). A number of modifications to the CAGE, such as the TWEAK (Chan, Pristach, Welte, & Russell, 1993), have produced improvements for some subpopulations. One variation on the CAGE replaces the question about being "Annoyed" with a question about "often driving *U*nder the influence of alcohol," thus creating the CUGE acronym. A recent study by Aertgeerts and colleagues (2000) suggests that this acronym may do a better job of identifying problematic college drinkers than the CAGE.

We believe the best screening tool for college students is the Alcohol Use Disorders Identification Test (AUDIT; Saunders, Aasland, Babor, De La Fuente, & Grant, 1993; see Appendix A). The AUDIT was developed by the World Health Organization to detect harmful alcohol consumption (as opposed to alcoholism). The AUDIT has been evaluated in many different populations around the world, including college students. The AUDIT contains 10 questions scored from 0 to 4 points (maximum score = 40): three questions on the amount and frequency of drinking, three questions regarding alcohol dependence, and four questions on alcohol-related problems. Among adults, a score of 8 or more indicates a high likelihood of an alcohol use disorder (Saunders et al., 1993).

Not surprisingly, the AUDIT typically outperforms other screening measures in college populations (Aertgeerts et al., 2000; Clements, 1998). Aertgeerts and colleagues (2000) found that a cut score of 6 provided the best discrimination for identifying problem drinking in a large group of European college students, and a similar result has been recently noted by Kokotailo and colleagues (2004) in an American sample. In an effort to make the process even briefer, researchers recently found that the first three items of the AUDIT (called the AUDIT-C), or in some cases just question #3 ("How often do you have six drinks or more on one occasion?"), identified alcohol problems among primary care patients in a Veterans Affairs hospital (Bradley et al., 2003). However, to our knowledge, this ultra-brief version of the AUDIT has not been tested with college populations.

Recommendations for Alcohol Screening

We recommend that college providers use the 10-question AUDIT to screen students for alcohol-related problems and use a score of 6 or more as an indicator of high-risk drinking and 8 or more as an indicator of a possible alcohol use disorder. (Further assessment, of course, would be necessary to confirm these indications.) The AUDIT is brief enough to be used in many contexts. In student health and counseling centers, we recommend that the AUDIT be included in the intake packet for all new patients.

If there is not time for the full 10-item AUDIT, we recommend asking the first three questions:

- *How often do you have a drink containing alcohol?*
- *How many drinks containing alcohol do you have on a typical day when you are drinking?*
- *How often do you have six drinks or more on one occasion?*

Decision rules for these three items in college students have not been tested to date. In the absence of data, we encourage the provider to use the student's answers to initiate a conversation about any alcohol-related difficulties and recommend at least brief advice if the student reports any episode of six or more drinks in the past month.

RELATED AREAS

Besides alcohol *involvement*, there are social and psychological factors that are often associated with alcohol use. For those interested in a more complete discussion of these areas, we suggest a review by Donovan (2004). Also, the BASICS manual (Dimeff et al., 1999) describes a number of assessments that can be useful for providing feedback to students about alcohol. We note just a few options here.

In a brief interaction, it is impossible to assess all the psychological and social factors related to alcohol. Even in a moderate-length interaction, options can be limited. However, with more available time, additional assessments can provide a broader understanding of the individual and supply information for providing feedback (see Chapter 6). Here we describe four dimensions that may be helpful in understanding young adult drinking: motivation, beliefs about alcohol's effects, drinking contexts, and family history of alcohol problems.

Motivation

Motivation or *readiness to change* describes a student's degree of interest in changing. As noted in Chapter 2, most college drinkers are either *precontemplators* or *contemplators*. Precontemplators do not see their alcohol use as a problem and rarely request help in changing behavior. Contemplators are wondering about or considering their options, but are not yet engaged in making changes. Therefore, a reasonable goal of an interaction may only be to raise concerns about drinking or to stimulate thoughts about change. Carey, Purnine, Maisto, and Carey (1999) have provided a thorough review of assessments related to assessment of readiness to change (see also Donovan, 2004). The key limitation for our purpose is that most scales designed to assess readiness, such as the University of Rhode Island Change Assessment (URICA; McConnaughy, Prochaska, & Velicer, 1983, 1989) and the Stages of Change Readiness and Treatment Eagerness Scale (SOCRATES; Miller & Tonigan, 1996), were developed with individuals either seeking or already in treatment for alcohol problems. Wording in these measures often refers to a recognition of problems related to alcohol and a desire to abstain from drinking. Because of this, these assessments can seem odd to many college students. They appear most useful for those students in formal counseling for alcohol problems or who have been referred for significant infractions (e.g., DUI).

A better scale to use with college students is the Readiness to Change Questionnaire (RTCQ; Rollnick, Heather, Gold, & Hall, 1992; see Appendix D). The RTCQ was developed for use in medical settings with individuals not seeking help for alcohol problems. It is brief (12 items), and the questions are more subtle—for instance, the word "problem" is avoided. Items include "My drinking is okay as it is," and "I am at the stage where I should think about drinking less alcohol."

For very brief interactions, the RTCQ is probably too lengthy. An alternative is the "Importance and Confidence Rulers" discussed in Chapter 5, which consists of two scaled questions about the importance and confidence of change.

- *On a scale of 1–10, how important is it for you to make a change in your drinking?*
- *On a scale of 1–10, how confident are you that you could change your drinking if you wanted to?*

The student's responses to these two questions give a quick indicator of two areas related to motivation—importance and confidence. The questions can also be worded differently, depending on what the clinician wants to assess. For instance, "How important is it for you to be safe when you drink?" is another alternative. In addition to gathering information about motivation, these questions can be part of the brief motivational exchange discussed in Chapter 5.

Alcohol Expectancies

Beliefs in alcohol effects describe people's expectations of what will happen when they drink. For instance, young adults commonly expect that alcohol will relieve anxiety, make parties more fun, and make them more attractive. Whether accurate or not, these beliefs are related to drinking. Knowing what a student expects from alcohol can also help the clinician understand reasons why he or she drinks and can reveal areas where students might feel less competent if they chose to make a change.

There are several options for assessing alcohol expectancies. We recommend the Comprehensive Effects of Alcohol scale (CEOA; Fromme, Stroot, and Kaplan, 1993; see Appendix E), which queries both positive and negative expectations about drinking. The CEOA asks students to identify ways they expect to feel after drinking—sexy, clumsy, sociable, and so on. We like the CEOA because it asks students to rate each effect in two ways: the likelihood that the effect will occur and how good or bad the student believes the effect will be. This combination allows the interviewer to tell whether the effects rated more likely to occur are also the ones rated most positively.

Drinking Context

Drinking context describes the social and psychological environments where drinking takes place (Thombs, Wolcott, & Farkash, 1997). Contexts vary depending on age, gender, living situation, and the function that alcohol serves at different times and places. There is some overlap here with the concept of alcohol expectancies, but drinking context scales can provide additional information about the things that surround drinking. For example, an individual may expect anxiety reduction from alcohol but drink only in social situations. A person like this is probably drinking for a different purpose than someone else who expects anxiety reduction but drinks alone.

Two different measures have been developed to assess drinking contexts. Using a group of high school students, Thombs and Beck (1994) developed a Social Context of Drinking Scale, with subscales assessing social facilitation, emotional pain, peer acceptance, family, sex seeking, and motor vehicle. O'Hare (1997b) offers a less comprehensive but more focused 23-item Drinking Context Scale, with three subfactors assessing convivial drinking, private intimate drinking, and negative coping. The O'Hare scale was developed with college students and appears to be the better option.

Family History

Family history of alcohol problems describes the extent to which a student has blood relatives who have had problems related to alcohol. Although family history of alcoholism is not a strong predictor of drinking during the college years (see Chapter 2), it can be a risk factor for alcohol problems later in life. The risk increases if the relatives are numerous, the same gender, and/or more closely related to the student. For this reason, we find that many students privately worry about their personal risk based on what they know about their families. Students want to know if they are at higher risk for developing alcohol problems not only currently, but over the next 10 or 20 years.

There are two brief techniques for assessing alcohol problems among relatives. One option is the Family Tree Questionnaire (FTQ; Mann, Sobell, Sobell, & Pavan, 1985), where students are presented with a picture of a family tree. After placing first- and second-degree relatives on the tree, a set of questions is asked about each person, indicating whether he or she experienced alcohol-related problems. If desired, the FTQ also provides a flexible method for assessing broader family trees and selected parts of families.

For briefer encounters, the student can be asked to give the number of blood relatives who are now, or have been in the past, problem drinkers or alcoholics:

> *Think about the number of your **blood relatives** who are now, or have been in the past, problem drinkers or alcoholics.*
>   *Number of parents?*   ____
>   *Number of brothers and sisters?*   ____
>   *Number of grandparents?*   ____
>   *Number of uncles and aunts?*   ____
>   *Number of first cousins?*   ____

The student receives two points for each first-degree relative (parent, brother, sister) and one point for each second-degree relative (grandparents, aunts, uncles, cousins). Using categories developed by the NIAAA (Miller, Zweben, DiClemente, & Rychtarik, 1995), the total number of points gives the student an estimated risk of low, medium, high, or very high (see Appendix G, Feedback Form, Section 3). Of course, even without an aggregate score, these assessments may provide interesting talking points about a student's family history.

CONCLUSION

In this chapter, we presented options for assessing drinking and related areas. Table 3.2 gives a summary of our recommendations. Given the central role of alcohol on campus, we strongly urge practitioners to regularly screen students who might be at risk. Almost any question about alcohol is better than nothing! A few key screening or consumption ques-

TABLE 3.2. Summary of Recommended Assessment Measures

	Time required		
Dimension	Brief (1–5 minutes)	Moderate (5–15 minutes)	Lengthy (15 minutes)
Consumption	Quantity–frequency Questions[a]	Daily Drinking Calendar[a]	Time Line Follow-Back (TLFB; Sobell et al., 1994)
Consequences	College Alcohol Problems Scale—Revised (CAPS-r; Maddock et al., 2001)[a]	Young Adult Alcohol Problems Screening Test (20-item YAAPST; Hurlbut & Sher, 1992)[a]	Same
Dependence			DSM Checklist (Forman et al., 2004; Hudziak et al., 1993)
Screening	Alcohol Use Disorders Identification Test (AUDIT-C; first three questions from the AUDIT; Bradley et al., 2003)[a]	AUDIT (Saunders et al., 1993)[a]	Same
Motivation	Importance and Confidence Rulers (Rollnick et al., 1999)[a]	Readiness to Change Questionnaire (RTCQ; Rollnick et al., 1992)[a]	Same
Expectations		Comprehensive Effects of Alcohol Scale (CEOA; Fromme et al., 1993)[a]	Comprehensive Effects of Alcohol Scale—Full Version
Context		Drinking Context Scale (DCS; O'Hare, 1997b)	Same
Family history	"Number of blood relatives" question (Miller et al., 1995)[a]	Same	Family Tree Questionnaire (FTQ; Mann et al., 1985)

[a]Measure reproduced in this book.

tions can be asked in less than three minutes. Unfortunately, our sense is that very few college providers ever ask students about their alcohol use. We suspect that many omit this important step not from a lack of awareness, but from a lack of time and knowledge of what to ask and perhaps from a fear about asking questions that might seem intrusive or rude. With all the important health issues vying for attention, we recognize that student service and health personnel are in a bind: too many questions about too many things in too little time. While we can't solve the larger problem of multiple demands on health services, we have tried to offer a few ways to quickly assess alcohol-related difficulties, as a prelude to a referral or brief intervention. Alcohol use can and should be discussed without judgment or embarrassment. Thus, we suggest an open, honest, and calm assessment style. The strategies we present in the next chapters can be helpful in setting a respectful tone for conversations about alcohol.

KEY POINTS

- Assessment helps us to better understand why a student drinks and tailor our approach to his or her needs. The assessment process need not take a long time—you can accomplish a lot with just a few basic questions.
- Planning assessments is important. Consider the purpose of the assessment and consider how much time you can realistically take.
- Limit questions that ask a student to report consistent patterns or average drinks over days, weeks, or months. As much as possible, ask about specific episodes of heavy drinking.
- When assessing drinking amount, be specific about the time frame. To estimate a peak BAC, ask about gender, weight, and time spent drinking.
- A detailed assessment of alcohol dependence or abuse is probably not necessary for working with most students, unless the student is showing other signs of risk. Rather, assessing alcohol-related consequences can be helpful in understanding the difficulties a student might be having related to alcohol.
- Brief screening tools, such as the AUDIT, can be useful for identifying students at special risk and for initiating a conversation about alcohol.
- Areas related to drinking, such as motivation, expectancies, drinking context, and family history are helpful in understanding why a student drinks, what reasons he or she might have to change, and what difficulties he or she might encounter in the future.

4

Style of the Interaction

OVERVIEW OF THE CHAPTER

As we mentioned in the introduction, this book presents a set of techniques derived from the counseling style of motivational interviewing (MI). While we rely on the framework of MI, many of the specific exercises are drawn from other approaches such as values clarification, skills training, relapse prevention, and cognitive-behavioral therapy. Although it is possible to conduct many of these techniques using another counseling style, we believe their effectiveness is greater when delivered using this evidence-based style.

This chapter describes the MI counseling style. We include this chapter for those who are new to the area or who want to brush up on their basic clinical skills. Why do we spend a whole chapter talking about style? One of the most interesting findings to emerge from clinical studies in recent years is that counseling style, almost irrespective of technique, is a predictor of client outcome. In fact, in many alcohol treatment studies, the variability among therapists is greater than the variability among treatment approaches. *How one conducts interviews is critical.* Thus, this chapter is intended to improve the reader's working knowledge of what we feel is the most effective way to have a conversation with college students about alcohol. Chapters 5, 6, and 7 suggest ways to structure different lengths of interactions—all are based on the style we outline in this chapter. For those not familiar with MI or who want to review the basics, we encourage an immersion in the logic of this approach.

WHO CAN TALK TO STUDENTS ABOUT ALCOHOL?

Almost all college drinkers interact with people who are concerned about their health and safety, such as healthcare workers, administrators, teachers, or resident assistants. In contrast, very few are referred to counselors who specialize in alcohol or drug abuse treatment. This means that nonspecialists will ultimately talk with many more college drinkers than specialized alcohol counselors will. Fortunately, there is good evidence that, under certain circumstances, individuals with relatively little counseling training can impact college student drinking (Fromme & Corbin, 2003; Larimer et al., 2001). A caveat: Although nonspecialists can be effective in many contexts, there are times when a trained specialist, such as a licensed counselor, social worker, or psychologist, is the appropriate one to conduct an intervention. We believe that it is best to refer a student to such a person when the student is at risk for immediate alcohol-related threats to safety or is suffering from mental health problems, abuse, or has thoughts of homicide or suicide. These sometimes serious problems should always be assessed and treated by a qualified professional.

DECONSTRUCTING THE STYLE OF THE INTERVIEW

Whether deciding to use alcohol, cut down, or quit, motivation plays a key role. In Chapter 2, we discussed the stages that people typically go through when they approach the possibility of change, and in Chapter 3, we presented a simple way to assess importance and confidence—two related factors. Here we make an additional point that the reader may have already guessed: *Motivation is malleable, rather than fixed.* Although a student may bring a certain motivational "profile" to an interaction, the way a provider conducts the conversation influences motivation from then on. Qualities of the provider, qualities of the student, and qualities of the interaction between them all influence change (or lack thereof) in the student's behavior. In short, *how* one talks to students about alcohol makes a difference.

Motivational interviewing, developed by William Miller and Stephen Rollnick (2002), is a client-centered, directive method for helping people explore and resolve ambivalence. By *client-centered*, they mean that each person has an innate capacity and responsibility for making choices in how to behave. Because of this, the provider works to clarify and amplify a student's own concerns about his or her behavior, without strongly imposing an agenda. Ultimately, the student must make the choice about whether or not to change. The task for the counselor is to create a set of conditions that facilitate this natural movement toward healthy change. By *directive*, they mean that the counselor picks certain statements and questions to steer the conversation in a particular direction. By *ambivalence*, they mean that most drinkers have mixed feelings about alcohol. Most students can list benefits and drawbacks of drinking, as well as of change. These mixed feelings need to be explored and, eventually, resolved.

Miller and Rollnick (2002) describe four general principles that underlie MI practice. These four principles are elements we strive for in our interactions with students.

1. *Express empathy.* The counselor actively listens to the student without judging, criticizing, or blaming. While the counselor may not agree with the student, he or she respects the student's point of view and autonomy. This active, empathic listening creates a "nest" where concerns can be freely explored.

2. *Develop discrepancy.* Motivation for change increases when individuals feel that there is a gap between where they are and where they would like to be. Depending on how the question is asked, most college drinkers will be able to identify ways that alcohol is affecting, or at risk for affecting, their schoolwork, health, or relationships or ways that drinking is inconsistent with other aspects of their life. These inconsistent feelings are "hooks" that the counselor uses to build motivation.

3. *Roll with resistance.* When considering a new behavior, it is natural to have competing "inner voices" that argue the pros and cons of the proposed change. Though ambivalent, the student might appear to have no interest in change or might be reluctant even to talk about it. Recognizing this, the counselor avoids arguing with the student. Rolling with resistance means finding other ways to respond when the counselor feels blocked or challenged.

4. *Support self-efficacy and talk for change.* Students must feel that they have some ability to implement changes before they will seriously consider them. The counselor supports this process through highlighting personal responsibility, identifying individual strengths, exploring past successes, and when appropriate, helping the student develop a plan for change.

Table 4.1 summarizes some of the more important differences between MI and other approaches that are often used in college settings. MI emphasizes listening and reflecting, personalizing information whenever possible, allowing students to express their own reasons for change, and collaborating on a change plan. MI does *not* advocate arguing with students, telling students what they "must" do, or insisting on a certain course of action. However different the approaches might look, we cannot overemphasize that the "spirit" is the critical distinction. The techniques in this book are designed to work when the counselor conveys empathy, respect, and positive expectations. In fact, as we mentioned at the beginning of this chapter, some believe that this interaction *style*, rather than the specific techniques used, best accounts for the remarkable track record of MI across a range of health behaviors (Miller, 2000; Hettema, Steele, & Miller, 2005).

WORKING WITH MOTIVATION

Just as there is tremendous variation in individual drinking, there is also tremendous variation in motivation to cut down or quit. In Chapter 3, we described ways to assess motivation. Here we discuss ways to use our understanding of an individual's motivational "profile" to make our interactions more effective. Picture motivation as having two dimen-

TABLE 4.1. Examples of MI-Consistent and MI-Inconsistent Behaviors

MI-consistent approach	MI-inconsistent approach
• Emphasis on listening, reflecting • More reflections than questions • Exploring ambivalence about change ("What have been some of the good things/not-so-good things?")	• Emphasis on talking, educating • More questions than reflections • Direct attempts to persuade ("Can't you see how your alcohol use is ruining your grades?")
• Personalized feedback ("Based on the amount you reported drinking, that puts you in the 95th percentile of U.S. college students.")	• General statistics or feedback ("Users have four times the amount of memory problems and sexual dysfunction compared to non-users.")
• Eliciting the student's own reasons for change ("It sounds like quitting would really save you money.").	• Telling the student why he or she should change ("Tests show that you have a problem with alcohol and need to do something about it.")
• Collaboration on a change plan ("What would you like to do differently to reduce your chance of blackouts?")	• Emphasis on taking action now ("You need to do something about this now, or you'll probably have another blackout.")

sions. One dimension is the *personal relevance* or *importance* of change. Consider the following three statements that a student might make about drinking.

1. *Things have gotten really bad. I've got to do something about my drinking.*
2. *My drinking can get out of hand sometimes, but it's not like I'm an alcoholic or anything.*
3. *Every college student I know drinks like me. There's nothing wrong with the way I drink.*

These statements reflect decreasing levels of interest in change. In the first statement, the student indicates that there is a problem and wants to change. In the second statement, the student has said that he or she is experiencing some consequences, but is still reluctant to change. The student is ambivalent—wanting to reduce use, but not seeing extreme "alcoholic" drinking patterns. The last statement expresses very little interest in change. The student does not see a problem, and may never have considered doing something different to be safer. In our experience, the last two patterns are the most common on college campuses. However, it is also quite possible, as we discuss below, that the student who states he or she has never considered change is actually ambivalent or undecided as to whether change might be beneficial

The second dimension of motivation involves beliefs about *confidence*. Some students would *like* to change, but think that they will not be *able* to. The student might be discouraged by past failures, an inhospitable environment, or other personal characteristics. Notice the subtle differences in the following statements:

1. *I know I should cut down on my drinking. I'll just have to leave the frat house during parties.*
2. *I know I should cut down on my drinking. It's just really hard living in a frat house.*
3. *I know I should cut down on my drinking. I just don't think it's possible living in a frat house.*

These statements reflect high desire but decreasing levels of confidence in change. The first and second statements tell us that the student thinks he *could* change. The first person even has a plan for dealing with a tempting situation. In contrast, the last person appears to *want* to change, but doesn't yet see a good solution.

Simplifying these importance and confidence ratings a bit, Table 4.2 summarizes motivational categories into which students might fall.

Let's examine each of the groups separately.

- *Group 1: These students have little interest in change, and don't think they could change even if they wanted to.* There are many reasons a student might fall into this motivational category. The first, of course, is that the student may not actually need to make a change in his or her drinking. Certainly, many students drink without being problem drinkers. Other students in this group have had some negative experiences, but do not see any real need to change. Because of this, it is important to use screening procedures like those described in Chapter 3 to take into account the amount that students are drinking, peak BACs, the degree to which they are experiencing drinking-related problems, and any evidence of alcohol dependence. Are there things the counselor sees, but the student doesn't? If so, screening questions can help a practitioner determine whether a student might benefit from a change. These students might also benefit from some of the strategies recommended for Group 3.
- *Group 2: These students want to change, but think any attempt will be doomed to failure.* High importance is a positive sign, but these students lack confidence. Some stu-

TABLE 4.2. Simplified Motivational Categories Based on Importance and Confidence

Confidence in ability	Importance of change	
	Low	High
Low	*Group 1*: See little reason to change, and don't think they could change even if they wanted to.	*Group 2*: Do not think they could change, even though it is important to them.
High	*Group 3*: See little reason to change, but think that they could change if they wanted to.	*Group 4*: Want to change, and are confident that they can.

dents are depressed and benefit from an intervention focused on mood. Some are isolated and benefit from social support. It can indeed be discouraging for students to think they will be all alone in their efforts or even ridiculed for trying. Other students are discouraged because of past failures to change. Students in this group often benefit from discussing a concrete plan, being reminded of the plan, and being held accountable through follow-up contact.

- *Group 3: These students think they could change, but it isn't a priority for them at this time*. In our experience, most college students fall into this category. Most are healthy, optimistic, and relatively protected from serious consequences. Drinking and some related consequences are part of the college package. When asked if they "could" change, most students say "Sure! If I wanted to." And when they do decide to change, most simply do it. They don't struggle, don't say a lot about it, and don't typically seek support. Students who *do* want support will ask a friend or family member. This is perhaps the biggest difference between the motivational profile of college drinkers and older drinkers. Most problem college drinkers are optimistic, but have not yet recognized the need for change (low importance, high confidence), while many older problem drinkers recognize the severity of their problem, but are worn down by past failures (high importance, low confidence). Students in this group benefit most from programs that encourage contemplation rather than specific plans or skills.

- *Group 4: These students are high in both importance and confidence and might be ready to talk about change*. On the surface, these students are showing all the signs of motivation, and it might be appropriate to proceed to a concrete plan of action.

- *Group 5*: We know that there is no Group 5 in the table, but we include it to denote another large group of *students who probably should not be concerned about drinking*. As described in Chapter 1, not all students drink heavily, and most heavy drinkers do so only occasionally. Likewise, many students do not experience significant consequences as a result of alcohol use. What consequences they do experience are outweighed by the benefits. We include these students in our motivational profiles to acknowledge their presence and because we frequently encounter them in intervention programs. Some are there because they are worried about a friend, a family member, or themselves (the "worried well"). Other students may have violated alcohol policy on a technicality (e.g., being in a room where alcohol is being consumed), even though they do not drink much. Other programs targeted at entire groups (e.g., fraternities or sororities) will no doubt include many of these low-risk, non-problem drinkers.

These rough groupings do not reflect the unique features of any single student, but they do allow us to make two suggestions related to motivation. First, *assess or listen for these dimensions*. Some counselors can get a sense of where a student is just by listening. Others find it helpful to ask the "importance–confidence" questions presented in Chapter 3. Second, *tailor plans and strategies based on importance and confidence*. The way you respond to students should vary based on these dimensions. Students in Group 1 (low interest, low confidence) must become more contemplative before they will attempt change. Many of the strategies described in this and subsequent chapters should be helpful for these kinds of students. Students in Group 2 (high importance, low confidence), although rarer, need approaches that target confidence. This kind of student might benefit by discussing and improving on past attempts, identifying a support network, or simply trying again. For students like this, strong warnings are not only unnecessary (importance already high), but actually can make them more worried and anxious about a decision they know they need to make. Students in Group 3 (low importance, high confidence)—in our opinion the most common type—profit most from consciousness-raising activities. These kinds of activities raise awareness of personal consumption (or the consumption of others), point out negative experiences or risks, and gently highlight ways that risky drinking conflicts with an individual's values, goals, or other behaviors. Students in Group 4 (high importance, high confidence) may need less help—the key may lie in developing a concrete plan or timeline for change. Finally, students in Group 5 can talk about ways to keep themselves safe, explore mixed feelings about others' use, and discuss ways to help friends who are having difficulties.

Sometimes a student scores high on both importance and confidence but still seems to be stuck. The importance–confidence model does have its limitations. Rollnick (1998) has suggested a variation on the "ready, willing, and able" analogy. A student who understands the need for change has fulfilled the "willing" element. Students confident in their abilities are "able." But for some, the combination of the two is not enough to tip the balance—they are still not "ready." What's missing? In some cases, it may be a matter of a concrete plan for implementing the new behavior: What's the timeline? If they will continue to drink, how much will they drink? Where will they be during high-risk situations? For these students, follow-up, accountability, and an open door are helpful. It may also be a matter of timing; that is, the student thinks some other time would be better. For these students, it can be helpful to discuss change in the hypothetical. How would the student make a change *if he or she wanted to* or *if the time were right*? The point is that, in describing aspects of a plan, students gain a better picture of what it might be like to make a change and take a step toward implementation.

CORE TECHNIQUES

In this section, we discuss basic techniques to gather information, create an empathic environment, and set the stage for talk about change. The first four, summarized by the acronym OARS (open-ended questions, affirmation, reflection, summary)—are similar to the reflective listening techniques used in client-centered counseling. The final technique, "elicit change talk," is more clearly directive. Reflective listening skills, though important, do not fully constitute the motivational interview. In MI, we clearly *do* have a direction— moving students toward reduced risk. If the student is taking risks, but not currently considering change, we want him or her to begin to think about it. If the student is ambivalent, we want to tip the balance toward safer decisions. And finally, if the student chooses to drink, we want him or her to be able to do so more safely. Through reflective listening, we attempt to minimize resistance of these goals, while at the same time gently paving a path in this direction.

Ask Open-Ended Questions

Rather than *telling* the student how he or she ought to feel or behave, the counselor focuses on *asking* the student how he or she is feeling, what concerns he or she has, and what changes he or she would like to make. This means that the student, rather than the counselor, does most of the talking. However, it is important to understand that the answers the student gives are, in part, determined by the questions we ask.

Specific, closed-ended questions are great when you know exactly what you are looking for: Do you mean this? How about this? Closed-ended questions are also good for getting people to talk *less*, because they limit responses. However, in motivational counseling interactions, it is generally better to ask *open-ended* questions—questions to which there are many possible answers. Closed-ended questions can be answered with a "yes" or "no" or with a number, for instance: "Do you drink frequently?" or "Are you worried about your drinking?" Both of these questions are dead ends. Fortunately, most closed-ended questions can easily be turned into open-ended questions. For instance, the question "Does this information surprise you?" is better said as "What do you think of this information?" Open-ended questions draw out thoughts and feelings from the student, rather than having the student confirm the thoughts of the interviewer, and keep the student talking.

Here are examples of a few open-ended questions:

- *What are your thoughts about alcohol here at the university?*
- *What part of your drinking most concerns you? What worries you about it?*
- *What do you make of this?*
- *In what situations do you drink the most? Where do you see the most drinking?*
- *In what situations is it hardest for you to stay sober?*

Here's an example of open-ended questions used to gather information about drinking:

COUNSELOR: Tell me a little bit about your drinking. *[open-ended question]*

STUDENT: I don't drink that much. I guess mostly on the weekends.

COUNSELOR: In what kind of situations? *[open-ended question]*

STUDENT: Well, I mean, parties are the big thing. I might have five or six beers when we party on Friday and Saturday night.

COUNSELOR: How about during the week? *[open-ended question]*

Open-ended questions pull for description, elaboration, and exploration. In addition to the information this student has given "on the surface" about drinking approximately 10 beers on the weekend, he has also volunteered information about the context in which he drinks (i.e., parties). He is mainly a social drinker.

Although questions can be an important tool for information-gathering, even the best ones tend to shift a person's attention. *People think in statements rather than questions.* This is why reflections (described below) are better than questions at facilitating a person's train of thought or gently directing it in a new course. A question also demands a response, which can highlight a subtle power differential between the asker and the responder. For these reasons, relative to reflective comments, use questions sparingly. Try not to ask two questions in a row, and never ask three in a row. The typical early pattern in an MI session is to ask an open-ended question and then follow the client's response with reflections, affirmation, and a summary.

Affirm

Social psychologists tell us that we form our opinions of people in the first few seconds of an interaction. While we may change our view of them in light of additional information, we usually adjust our initial impression rather than toss it out and start from scratch. This is one reason we affirm a student early through statements of appreciation and understanding.

- *Thanks for being on time. I appreciate you coming in today.*
- *Those are some really good ideas.*
- *Thanks for hanging in there. I know this isn't what you had planned to do with your Saturday.*
- *Even though things got screwed up, it seems to you that you were trying to do what was best.*

Look for opportunities to affirm the student in a sincere way. Affirmations build a good counseling "nest" in which a student can feel safe speaking honestly and sharing concerns. Affirmations also support the self-efficacy that is necessary for change. Here's an example:

STUDENT: Sure, I drink some, but so does everyone else. Our sorority does a pretty good job of taking care of each other. We let another sister know when she's had too much to drink, and if we go out for an evening, we always come back as a group.

COUNSELOR: Sounds like you really take care of each other. *[affirmation]*

STUDENT: Well, yeah, that's what sorority life is about. Looking out for your sisters.

COUNSELOR: It's obvious that you've thought a lot about this. What other things do you do to make sure you stay safe? *[affirmation, open-ended question]*

These sincere praises have a number of positive effects. First, if the student feels reinforced for her comment, she is more likely to make similar comments and elaborate on what she has said. Second, the student becomes surer that you are an ally rather than a foe and is more likely to talk with you about potential concerns. Third, affirmations raise the student's self-efficacy or belief in her own abilities. Successes in small things make successes in large things more possible.

Here's another example:

STUDENT: I guess I could pace myself on Friday nights.

COUNSELOR: Good suggestion. How would you do that? *[affirmation, open-ended question]*

STUDENT: Well, nobody bugs the designated driver to drink. I think if I agreed to be the designated driver more often, it would be easier to drink less. I think I'd feel good helping out too.

COUNSELOR: Yeah, I think you would too. Great idea! *[affirmation]*

Any verbal steps the student takes toward change, however small, should be recognized. Although the student has not sworn off drinking, he or she has taken a step in a positive direction. Also note that in this example (as in all our examples), the counselor avoids pejorative phrases such as "addiction," "alcoholism," or "drinking problem." In addition to being probably inappropriate descriptors, such terms can sound critical and judgmental to many young people. Rather, whenever possible, we recommend that language be nonjudgmental. For instance, instead of the word "problems," we might suggest "difficulties," "downsides," or a more general word like "issues."

Listen Reflectively

Beginning counselors often underestimate the power of an aptly placed reflection. In truth, quite a lot of good counseling is simply restating to the client what he or she feels, thinks, or has said. Reflections have important purposes: to let the student know that *you understand what is being said*, to *underscore something* a student has said, and to *diffuse hostile emotions*.

When we reflect, we engage in a kind of hypothesis testing. Because there are steps between what the student means and what we *think* he or she means, we reflect to determine whether our hypotheses are correct. As Figure 4.1 illustrates, our hypothesis can go wrong if (1) the speaker does not say what he or she means, (2) we hear the speaker incorrectly, or (3) we misinterpret the speaker's meaning.

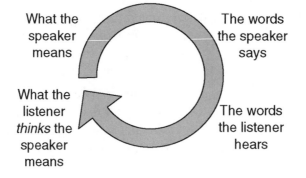

FIGURE 4.1. Reflective listening process.

Since reflections are a hypothesis about what a person is thinking or feeling, the common subject word is "you":

- *So you/you're . . .*
- *It looks like you . . .*
- *You've noticed that . . . You're also worried that . . .*
- *Let me see if I have this right. You . . .*
- *You're surprised/angry/confused/frustrated . . .*

Consistent with an active style of listening, the counselor listens to the student and reflects back what he or she is saying, both verbally and nonverbally. *Simple* reflections restate or paraphrase what the student has said.

COUNSELOR: (*presenting feedback to a female student*) Based on the assessment information you gave, that puts you at about the 97th percentile of female college students in terms of your drinking. [*gives information*]

STUDENT: (*looking surprised*) Whoa! That's really up there.

COUNSELOR: You're surprised that it's that high. [*reflection*]

STUDENT: Yeah, that seems a little . . . I don't know where you got your numbers, but there's no way that I am up that high.

COUNSELOR: It's pretty hard to believe. [*reflection*]

Reflections are like the narrator's voice in a movie. The narrator cuts through the dialogue to explain what the character is *really* thinking. Like a good narrator, most good reflections do not parrot the person's exact words, but push a bit forward, in a way that Miller and Rollnick (2002) call "continuing the paragraph." By this, they mean that the best reflections are something that the student might have said if he or she continued to talk. More than just an echo of the student's voice, reflections move *just beyond* what the student has said to give momentum to the conversation. In this example, the counselor reflects the student's emotional reaction to the feedback. Although the student didn't use the word "surprised," it's clear that surprise was the emotion she was feeling. The student may have also given some nonverbal cues such as widened eyes or an opened mouth. Had she continued to talk about the way she was feeling, she might very well have used a phrase similar to the one the counselor chose. When the student begins to dispute the results, the counselor restates her reaction. The tension means that the student is thinking about the information. The information surprises the student, and the reflection underscores this tension.

A more complicated reflection may highlight mixed feelings. These *double-sided* reflections are appropriate when a student feels two ways about something or has articulated two sides of an issue. Double-sided reflections call attention to ambivalence:

- *On the one hand, you feel like your drinking is risky, but on the other hand, you don't see anyone else who seems to be concerned about it.*
- *So, your girlfriend/parents/friends worry about your drinking, but you don't see it the same way.*
- *You can't imagine being at a party without drinking, but at the same time you have a sense that you should be able to party without alcohol.*

Here's an example of reflections used to highlight a negative aspect of drinking, as well as ambivalence about change.

COUNSELOR: I see from your assessment that you have some questions related to your alcohol use. Which of these has been on your mind lately? *[open-ended question]*

STUDENT: When I party the night before a soccer game, I really pay for it the next day.

COUNSELOR: So the thing that concerns you is the way it's affecting your soccer performance. *[reflection]*

STUDENT: Yeah, that's the main thing. I mean, I'm not an alcoholic or anything. My grades have always been really good.

COUNSELOR: Okay, so on the one hand, you like to have a good time and hang out with your friends the night before a game, but on the other hand, you sometimes end up drinking more than you wanted, and you really pay for it the next day. *[double-sided reflection]*

The counselor initiates the conversation with an open-ended question and then reflects the student's response. The student's reply tells us that he is ambivalent. He is stuck, at odds, in a pickle, having mixed feelings. In this case, since the student uses the word "alcoholic," it may be that he is conflicted because his drinking doesn't fit either of the extreme pictures he has in his head. He is neither the "safe" social drinker nor the alcoholic. He's somewhere in the middle. He may also be ambivalent because he has not yet decided what, if anything, he would like to do about his drinking. For many students, the decision to change is a complicated one that involves social, physical, and financial factors. Is there a roommate or girlfriend involved? What will he do with the case of beer he bought yesterday? How would he fit in if he didn't drink with his friends? Before committing to something new, this student may need time to decide whether, all things considered, it will be worth it.

Table 4.3 illustrates another use of reflective comments in a slightly different context—when students are angry or resistant. These reflections let the student know that you understand what they are saying.

Since we are not using direct attempts to persuade, speak to disarm, not to overpower. One important task, especially early in an interaction, is to let the student know that you understand his or her point of view. Here's an example of a particularly difficult session with a student referred by campus police for underage drinking.

> COUNSELOR: I'd like to understand a little about your drinking. What brings you here? *[open-ended question]*
>
> STUDENT: It wasn't my fault! We were just hanging out, and someone had a beer can. I took my one-and-only drink when the officer came around the corner, and bam! here I am.
>
> COUNSELOR: So it seems unfair. *[reflection]*
>
> STUDENT: Yeah! This campus has a hundred rapes a year, and they bust me for having a sip of beer? It doesn't make any sense!
>
> COUNSELOR: It seems to you like the police should be spending their time on other things. *[reflection]*
>
> STUDENT: Yeah, this campus sucks.
>
> COUNSELOR: Okay, you have to be here, even though it's not what you'd rather be doing. It pisses you off. *(pause)* So, I'm wondering, since we have to be here, what

TABLE 4.3. "Rolling with" Resistant Comments

Resistant statement	Possible reflection
"I'm not the one with the problem!"	"You don't feel like you have a problem."
"Who are you to tell me what to do?"	"You don't feel like I can understand where you're coming from."
"I like drinking!"	"Drinking has some positive aspects for you."
"I don't know why I'm here. This whole thing is stupid!"	"You're frustrated with having to be here!"

could we talk about during this time that *would* be helpful to you? *[reflection, open-ended question]*

Many counselors, even experienced ones, would have a hard time talking to this student without "biting" in reaction to his provocative comments. It wasn't his fault! The police unfairly targeted him! Other students have worse problems! The student has clearly baited the counselor in an attempt to derail the discussion. The counselor *could* argue with the student about the campus environment, the role of the police, etc., but these issues are beside the point. The counselor's task is to help the student examine his or her thoughts and feelings about alcohol to see whether a change would be beneficial. In this example, the counselor disarms the student's anger by validating the emotion. In most cases, a student only needs to know that someone else knows that he feels angry or reluctant or wronged.

Even though the counselor should fairly reflect what the student has said, reflection can be *selective* to some extent. That is, the counselor can reflect certain aspects of what the student is saying or ignore other aspects to guide the conversation in a particular direction. For instance, consider this complex statement:

My girlfriend has really started to nag me about my drinking, but that's okay. She nags me about a lot of stuff.

The student is saying three things: (1) His girlfriend is worried about his drinking; (2) her worry does not concern him; and (3) she worries about lots of things. If you were to use a reflective comment or ask for elaboration, to which element would you respond? If the goal is to encourage the student to examine his drinking, it's probably best to respond to the first element because it will get the student talking (if only in the abstract) about potential problems. Following element 2 will get the student talking about his lack of concern for his girlfriend's opinions, while element 3 initiates a conversation about the girlfriend's annoying style of expressing concern. *Where the conversation goes depends on which aspect you reflect.* In this example, only the first element initiates a conversation that is likely to be fruitful down the line.

- A reflective statement summarizes the girlfriend's concerns: *Your girlfriend has some concerns about your drinking.*
- An open-ended question asks for elaboration on the girlfriend's concerns: *What concerns does your girlfriend have about your drinking?*

Summarize

Summaries are larger reflections that underscore several comments the student has made or a theme that has appeared. Summaries show that you have been listening, point out a theme, and encourage the student to elaborate further. In addition to giving a fair synopsis of what the student has said, the counselor can choose to stress certain aspects (e.g., concerns, confidence because of past successes). If there was resistance or ambivalence during the session, this should be reflected as well. Some summaries call attention to a theme that has emerged, for instance when a student has made several similar statements in a row. Other summaries contrast what a student said at the beginning of the session with what was said at the end of the session. If appropriate, a summary can be followed by an open-ended request (e.g., "What else?").

- [Summary of drinking demography] *Let me see if I have this right. You've said that you drink about 10 drinks per week, mainly on the weekends and sometimes on Wednesdays and Thursdays. There have been some bumps in the road, but in general, drinking has not really been a problem for you. You think that, in the long run, your drinking will go way down because it doesn't really fit your ideas of what it would be like to have a family. But for now, it sort of does fit into your experience. Is that about right?*
- [Summary of reasons for wanting to cut down] *Okay, so the worst part of the increased drinking this semester seems to be the effect on your schoolwork. You mentioned that while you like to party, you also get tired, and this affects your ability to study for classes. You also mentioned that you've already had to drop a course because you missed too many classes. What else?*
- [Summary reflecting ambivalence] *You sound stuck! On the one hand, you've always thought that getting drunk was just part of the college experience. It was something you were supposed to do to spread your wings. On the other hand, if your drinking puts you at the 90th percentile of college drinkers, that means you are drinking more than the vast majority of college students. It's confusing. What thoughts come next as you think about this?*

Another kind of summary is used when transitioning from one section to another or to end an interaction. In contrast to summaries that keep the session moving, these summaries close a section and announce what will come next.

It looks like we are about out of time, and I want to try to pull together what we've talked about so far. You came in very aware of some issues related to your drinking. You said that it was very important for you to make a change because you're having trouble staying focused during the day. You were also pretty confident that you could cut down. We talked about what you might like to do about it, and you thought that the most helpful thing would be to keep track of your drinking over the next week and check in with me a couple more times. Is that about it? Did I miss anything?

The counselor reviews the material discussed and ends the session. As discussed above, pejorative terms like "alcoholic," "addiction," and even "problem" are avoided unless specifically used by the student, and he or she is given the opportunity to correct or clarify the summary. If the student returns for another session, it might also be appropriate to begin with a summary of what was discussed during the last session.

Elicit Change Talk

The OARS skills in the previous sections are critical to motivational interviewing. However, because MI is a *directive* therapy, we also work to maximize certain kinds of statements. "Change talk" is a broad term that refers to all kinds of talk about change. It might include dissatisfaction with present behavior, what things would look like as a result of different behaviors, plans (even hypothetical ones) to change, or a verbal commitment. In one very interesting study (Amrhein, Miller, Yahne, Palmer, & Fulcher, 2003), an analysis of speech during a single counseling session showed that clients with the best outcome were those who expressed an increasing amount of "commitment" language—one type of change talk—over the course of the session, particularly near the end of the session. There is experimental data too. In other studies, MI doubles the amount of change talk relative to other kinds of therapy (Miller, Benefield, & Tonigan, 1993).

The phrase "I know what I believe when I hear myself say it" rings true. People are much more likely to implement a behavior if they feel they authored the idea. For this reason, the student is the primary source for finding answers and solutions. Our discussion of open-ended questions, affirmations, reflections, and summaries (OARS) presents several techniques that *minimize resistance*, or the likelihood that students will express language opposite to change. But we can also encourage talk in support of change through carefully phrased reflections and comments and by asking for elaboration on certain things the student says.

Recognizing and reinforcing change talk is an important skill for counselors. Change statements generally fall into one of four categories (adapted from Miller & Rollnick, 2002):

- *Disadvantages of the status quo (if drinking in a high-risk way)*. These statements acknowledge that there are drawbacks or disadvantages to the present behavior. The student need not admit that there is a "problem," but only that there are some undesirable aspects of his or her drinking.
- *Advantages of change*. These statements recognize the advantages of behavior change. While the first category focuses on the not-so-good things about the present behavior, this one focuses on the good things to be gained through change.
- *Optimism for change*. These statements indicate that the student believes he or she has the skills, supports, or abilities to change, either in the abstract (e.g., "I could") or the concrete (e.g., "I can").
- *Intention to change*. These statements show that the balance of motivation has shifted. The student moves from talking about change in the abstract to making verbal commitments (e.g., "I will").

To elicit change talk, the counselor might ask the student to elaborate on his or her own reasons for change, the advantages of change, or confidence in his or her ability. When a student makes a change statement, immediately reflect and ask for elaboration. In Chapter 6, we present structured exercises that can increase the likelihood that students will make change statements. More generally, however, questions like the ones below make change statements more likely.

Ask about present concerns:

- *What makes you think this is an issue?*
- *What are some of the downsides to your drinking?*
- *Can you give me an example of that? What was that like?*
- *What else?*

Ask about the past:

- *Tell me about the last time you got really drunk. What happened?*
- *Give me an example of a time when things were going really well . . . What was that like?*
- *What were things like before you began drinking?*
- *How was last semester different (when you weren't drinking)?*

Ask about the future:

- *How do you think your drinking will change in the long run?*
- *Suppose things don't change. Where do you think you'll be in 5 years down the road?*
- *Where do you think you'll be in 10 years? What will your drinking look like?*
- *If you did decide to change, what would the change look like?*

Ask about change:

- *What are you thinking you'd like to do about this?*
- *Where does this leave you in terms of your drinking?*
- *Now that you've shared these concerns, what would you like to do about them?*
- *What's your plan? What's your policy about . . . ?*

Although it can sometimes be difficult to know which statements to reflect, here is a general rule: *Early in an interaction, if appropriate, ambivalence should be reflected, while later, after exploring ambivalence, change talk should be more attended to.* We cannot leave this discussion of the elicitation of change talk without one important reminder: Do not lose your primary reflective position. Many counselors, once instructed to ask certain types of questions, quickly forget to reflect and summarize what they are hearing. Questions should be used sparingly and only in the context of liberal affirmations, reflections, and summaries.

WHAT COMES NEXT?

The skills above—open-ended questions, affirmations, reflections, summaries, and eliciting change talk—are the building blocks of MI. Of course, blocks are only one component of a well-built structure. There can be great variety in how one links the blocks together. Having used these techniques for several years, we are not surprised that Miller and Rollnick (2002) ultimately define MI as a "style" or a "way of being with people." When one is really listening to students—communicating and understanding, while still supporting ideas and plans for change—technique is eclipsed by style. In the chapters that follow, we describe techniques for reducing resistance, stimulating contemplation, and developing discrepancy. In our opinion, however, the MI style is the foundation on which the techniques are built.

KEY POINTS

- MI is a person-centered, directive approach that is collaborative, reflective, and evocative. Express empathy, develop discrepancy, roll with resistance, and support self-efficacy.
- Client behavior is, in part, a reaction to counselor behavior. Resist the urge to "fix" the student by taking up the positive side of change. Rather, listen and speak in a way that reduces resistance and encourages the student to voice his or her own reasons for change.
- Motivation to change is made up of at least two components: importance and confidence. Recognize and tailor your approach to each student's unique motivational profile.
- What looks like lack of motivation is often ambivalence. Since both voices are already in the student, try to engage a student's inner voice for change.
- Use reflective listening techniques (open-ended questions, affirmation, reflection, and summary) to gather information, create an empathic environment, and set the stage for talk about change.
- Reflections are better than questions at steering a motivational train of thought. When possible, use more reflections than questions.
- Language during an interaction predicts later change. Because of this, encourage change talk by asking the student to elaborate on the disadvantages of current behavior, benefits of change, optimism, and commitment to new behavior.

5

Brief Individual Interactions
ADVICE AND CONSULTATION

OVERVIEW OF THE CHAPTER

In this chapter, we describe ways to engage students in conversations about alcohol through brief and opportunistic interactions. By *brief*, we mean less time than the traditional 50-minute counseling session, though in some instances it may mean only a few minutes. By *opportunistic*, we mean that the encounter may be unplanned—in doctors' offices, waiting rooms, classrooms, or administrative offices. Alcohol may not be the stated reason for the conversation. In fact, drinking may be the farthest thing from the student's mind. Brief interactions about alcohol can occur as part of a routine health examination, before prescribing a medication that interacts with alcohol, or in response to presenting problems that may be linked to alcohol or drugs. Slightly longer interactions can occur after a referral for alcohol-related difficulties or just in informal conversations with faculty or administrative staff. The commonality is that the provider takes advantage of a situation where a brief conversation about alcohol might be helpful to the student. We include this chapter because these kinds of interactions are very common on college campuses and because they have a great and underutilized potential to reduce alcohol-related harm. Because there is less research on these briefest interventions, this chapter draws heavily on alcohol intervention research in medical settings (Dunn, 2003; Emmen et al., 2004; World Health Organization, 1996).[1]

We start the chapter by discussing ways to broach the subject of drinking without raising resistance. We then describe ways to use MI strategies in relatively brief spans of time. We finish by offering a few strategies and techniques that are sometimes helpful in brief

---

[1]Many of the strategies in this chapter have been adapted from Rollnick and colleagues (1999). For those who work specifically in medical settings, we also recommend Banyard (2002), or Stuart and Lieberman (2002).

encounters, including two sample interactions organized around available time: *brief advice* (3–10 minutes) and *behavioral consultation* (10–30 minutes).

WHAT MOTIVATES PEOPLE IN BRIEF INTERACTIONS?

When trying to motivate someone quickly, it can be tempting to provide strong suggestions and advice. In very brief encounters, we may indeed be relegated to advice giving. However, the problem with well-intentioned advice is that people don't often take it. People are much more likely to adopt opinions and behaviors that they believe they have personally authored, as opposed to something that seems to come from another person. Not only do people generate more practical ideas on their own, but there also seem to be ownership factors that result from hearing oneself voice an opinion. *People become more committed to that to which they give voice.* For this reason, quick statements of advice are rarely optimal for persuading. However, at the same time, some very brief interactions do have an impact on drinking (World Health Organization, 1996). As we have already mentioned, when the effective elements are parsed out of the interventions, the active ingredients seem to have less to do with the information conveyed and more to do with the *style* of the interaction—concern, empathy, and reflective listening. This is true for brief, as well as longer interactions. Therefore, whenever possible, through our compassionate style, active listening, and use of key questions and reflections, we attempt to get the student to voice his or her *own* reasons to change. As with the longer interactions we describe in the next chapter, briefer interactions hinge on these principles. Indeed, *providing good information badly* may be the most common error in brief interactions.

At this point, it may be helpful to mention some of the ways that brief interventions differ practically from longer interventions. First, in brief interventions there is obviously less "talk time." This means less time for open-ended questions, affirmations, reflections, and summaries. Likewise, there may be very little time for structured counseling techniques like motivational feedback. Longer interventions look more like counseling sessions, while shorter interventions look more like conversations. Second, a brief intervention may be less structured. The environment may be noisy and chaotic, the topic of alcohol may be totally unexpected by the student, and the practitioner may have a range of issues that he or she must address in addition to alcohol use. Third, in brief interventions there may be less overt attention to a student's ambivalence. In shorter interactions, ambivalence becomes an assumption of the conversation, rather than the focus of specific techniques.

BROACHING THE SUBJECT

The first task in a brief intervention is broaching the subject of drinking. If the student expects the interaction—as may be the case with referrals to residence hall or student health personnel—he or she may already have ideas about what the interaction will be like. In situations like this, it is important to assure the student that you are not there to lecture, cajole, or argue. (The student may not believe you, but say it anyway!) You hope to have a conversation about drinking that might be helpful, but any decision to change will be left to the student.

If the student *does not* expect the interaction—as may be the case when a problem is first noticed by faculty, staff, or health personnel—he or she may be caught off guard. This makes the task doubly difficult. Not only must the provider quickly broach the subject, but he or she must do so without making the transition seem abrupt and thereby raising the student's defensiveness. Below we suggest two ways to transition a conversation to a discussion about drinking. The first way is to share your concerns about the student's drinking. The second way is to provide an opportunity for the student to raise his or her own concerns about alcohol.

Sharing Your Concerns

To raise the issue of alcohol or drug use, one simple format is to express your concern ("I noticed that . . .") and ask for permission to provide information or advice ("I wonder if . . .").

- [Resident advisor; roommate reported that student has been skipping classes and often seems hung-over.] *I noticed that you have been having some trouble with your classes lately. I wonder if I could talk to you about what's going on.*
- [Sorority mother; sorority pledge has rapidly accelerated drinking.] *I noticed that things seemed to get a little out of hand at the party last night, and that concerns me because I really want you to join the house. I wonder if I could ask you some questions in confidence about your drinking.*
- [Nurse at student health center; student endorses AUDIT question "8" (blackouts) on intake packet.] *I noticed that on the intake packet, you said that there have been a few times in the last year where you were unable to remember what happened while you were drinking. I wonder if I could provide you with some information about what might be going on.*

In expressing concern, use clear language and specific examples. As discussed in the last chapter, we recommend avoiding pejorative terms such as "problem." Words like this tend to make the student more defensive and are, in our opinion, unnecessary. Simply share what you have noticed and provide information. Each of the preceding dialogues might be followed by a brief alcohol screening (see Chapter 3), advice (see Providing Advice and Suggestions section, Chapter 5, p. 63, or the Importance and Confidence Rulers (see Importance and Confidence Rulers section, Chapter 5, p. 67.

Exploring the Student's Own Concerns

A second way to broach the subject is to give the student an opportunity to express his or her own concerns about alcohol. For instance, student health or counseling offices might include a checklist in the intake assessment, "Things I Would Like to Talk to My Doctor About." Items on this list might include alcohol and drug use, smoking, depression, medication concerns, problems with schoolwork, and other lifestyle difficulties common to college students. If a student completes the checklist along with other intake assessments, the completed form can be given to a doctor, nurse, or counselor. The information becomes a springboard for discussing concerns with the student. Another method is for the provider directly to ask students what concerns *they* have about their alcohol use or what difficulties they have experienced as a result of drinking. Finally, with slightly more time, the "Good Things, Not-So-Good Things" strategy we discuss in Chapter 6 can be helpful in raising difficulties the student has had related to drinking. In short, the activity involves asking students to name some of the things they *like* about alcohol (e.g., "What are some of the good things about your drinking?"), followed by some of the *drawbacks* (e.g., "What have been some of the not-so-good things?"). In addition to highlighting ambivalence about drinking, this question pair can move students away from a hard pro-alcohol stance into one that is more mixed.

- [Physician at health clinic] *It seems that alcohol might be an issue here. I'd really like to hear your perspective.*
- [Counselor] *In your experience, what have been some of the not-so-good things about drinking?*
- [Resident advisor] *It sounds like you have expressed some concerns to others about alcohol use. What are your concerns? Your thoughts and impressions are really important to me.*

PROVIDING ADVICE AND SUGGESTIONS

As we mentioned, those who have only brief interactions with students may be limited to providing advice or suggestions. Because suggestions are sometimes helpful, the temptation for the provider is to provide *unsolicited* recommendations in an attempt to solve the problem quickly. This information is often phrased in imperative (e.g., "You must . . .") or prescriptive (e.g., "You should . . .") terms. Fear induction (e.g., "If you don't . . . you might . . .") is sometimes part of the process. However, the risk is that this strong advice-giving stance may make some students more resistant to the idea of change.

The spirit of the interaction is critical. A warm and empathic style will carry advice much further than an authoritative stance. A warm, caring attitude makes students more likely to listen to the message, follow up on the advice, and contact the provider for further information. In addition to the underlying spirit, other factors make it more likely that students will consider the advice:

- *Ask for permission before providing advice* (e.g., "Would it be okay if I gave you some information about . . . ?").
- *Preface advice with permission to disagree* (e.g., "This may or may not apply to you, but . . .").
- *Give a small amount of essential information.* Many students may be confused and overwhelmed by information, and we don't want to reduce the effectiveness of our core message by placing too many demands on them. Rather, give bite-sized chunks of clear information or suggestions.
- Rather than giving a one-size-fits-all solution, *give several options* for how the student might address the difficulty (e.g., "There are several things that students in your position tend to find helpful").
- *Negotiate a plan of action.* In truth, students have many options—reducing consumption, avoiding high-risk situations, or simply agreeing to think about change. Chapter 6 gives a list of benchmarks that are sometimes helpful in choosing a drinking goal. All (or none) of these may be viable courses of action, depending on the student.

One way to structure advice is to provide some information, while still eliciting the student's opinions and ideas. Rollnick and colleagues (1999) suggest the "elicit–provide–elicit" (E-P-E) format as a way to convey information to individuals at risk. In this technique, the student is first asked to describe what he or she knows about a particular health behavior or what concerns or questions he or she has (*elicit*). Next, the counselor gives clear, nonjudgmental advice (*provide*), using specific examples if available. Finally, the student is asked what he or she would like to do about the behavior (*elicit*). For instance:

Elicit readiness and interest.
    What do you know about the effects of alcohol on . . . ?
    What concerns do you have about . . . ?

Provide clear information or feedback.
    The results of your tests suggest that . . .
    What happens to some people is that . . .
    As your doctor/counselor/RA, I strongly urge you to. . . .

Elicit the student's interpretation or reaction.
    What do you think?
    How do you think you might . . . ?

For instance, in the following dialogue, a health center nurse uses the E-P-E format to structure a brief interaction with a student who has been referred to the student health center.

> COUNSELOR: Thanks for completing the intake assessments. I noticed that you reported you've had some blackouts while drinking, and I wonder if I could ask you some questions about those. [affirmation, asks for permission]
>
> STUDENT: I guess that's okay.
>
> COUNSELOR: What do you know about the causes of blackouts? [elicits request for information]
>
> STUDENT: I don't know . . . It's probably not good. But I heard that a lot of students sometimes have them, so I figure it couldn't be that bad.
>
> COUNSELOR: Actually, blackouts can be a serious problem for a couple of reasons. From a physiological standpoint, it's an indicator that alcohol is coming into the system faster than the brain can handle. Because of the memory loss, people are at much greater risk of injuring themselves or others. So for some people it can be a real problem. [provides information]
>
> STUDENT: Hmm.
>
> COUNSELOR: So, where does this leave you? I am interested in your thoughts. [elicits reaction]

E-P-E reverses the usual advice hierarchy by allowing the student to do most of the talking—it is *student centered*. The typical (and we think less effective) method is to start by providing information, allow the student to react, and then correct the student's viewpoint or make additional suggestions on the way out of the conversation. In contrast, the E-P-E format allows the student to voice concerns and encourages better synthesis of the material. We also recommend the E-P-E format when drinking is clearly contraindicated—for instance, in advising pregnant women or those with other health conditions against drinking.

Responding to Direct Requests for Advice

What do *you* think I should do? Students do sometimes ask for advice. Students may ask for your opinion on what they should do or how they should do it. In instances like this, it can be appropriate to provide suggestions. However, even when the student has clearly asked for help, we still recommend proceeding with caution. Less interested students may ask for advice so that they can counter suggestions and leave the interaction even more convinced that their case is hopeless. Students may also make self-defeating statements. We sometimes hear statements like "There's just nothing I can do. It's impossible to live in a frat house and not drink." It can be very tempting to bombard the student with suggestions. But rushing to provide suggestions can trap you into an argument—you provide solutions while the student refutes them. A better format, we believe, is either to *ask the student what he or she thinks* or *offer a menu of alternatives*. In both cases, leave the onus for change with the student. For instance:

- *What have you thought of? What might work for you?*
- *Well, you're the one that ultimately will have to make the choice. What would you recommend to another student in your situation?*
- *There are a few things that students in your situation sometimes find helpful . . .* [provide a short list]. *Which of these do you think will work for you?*

The last phrase (one of our favorites) can be extremely useful. Notice the phrasing. First, we have provided a menu of options for the student, which makes it more likely that the student will find one that suits him or her. This also makes it more likely that the student will begin to *own* the idea. If picked from a personal menu, rather than advised by someone else, the student did indeed have a hand in generating the strategy. Second, by following with an open-ended question, we again make it more likely that the student will give an affirmative response. In our opinion, the closed-ended alternative ("Do you think any of these will work for you?") makes it more likely that the student will simply say, "No, none of these will work."

Once the student has responded, immediately reinforce and follow up:

- *So that might work for you. How would (will) you go about that?*
- *That sounds like a really good idea. Tell me more.*
- *What would (will) that look like?*
- *Great! What's your plan?*

EXPLORING CHANGE IN THE ABSTRACT

Despite our efforts to increase interest and readiness, many students will leave the brief interaction unconvinced. For those students who are drinking in a risky fashion, our goal may be simply to get the student to think about whether a change might be beneficial. A substantial decision (or series of small decisions) may happen at some point in the future as a result of this raised awareness, but the provider will see little overt movement during the interaction.

For the reluctant student, one useful strategy is to discuss change in the *hypothetical* rather than the concrete. This gives the student permission to explore the possibility of change without having to commit to a specific course of action. Basically, this involves discussing actions that a student might take *if he or she wanted to*, that is, behaviors conditional on desire (Table 5.1). The student can freely explore plans, decisions, or behaviors without having to commit to any of them.

TABLE 5.1. Change in the Abstract

Conditional statement	Plan of action
"If you wanted to . . ."	"How would you do it?"
"If you decided you wanted to . . ."	"How would you go about it?"
"If the time were right . . ."	"What would you do?"

Here's an example of a student who recognizes that drinking has been largely responsible for a deterioration in his or her grades but isn't ready to commit to a course of action. The provider asks about change in the hypothetical and gently reinforces concrete plans and statements.

COUNSELOR: So, on the one hand, you recognize that partying makes it hard for you to keep up your grades, but on the other hand, you're not sure whether it makes sense to change your drinking. *[double-sided reflection]*

STUDENT: Well, yeah. I mean, I know things get a little out of hand sometimes, but I like to have fun on the weekend. My class just kind of gets in the way . . .

COUNSELOR: Well, let me ask you this. If you decided to cut down, how would you do it? *[hypothetical open-ended question]*

STUDENT: I guess I would have to decide ahead of time that I either wouldn't drink on Sunday night, or I'd set a limit.

COUNSELOR: How would that work? *[open-ended question]*

In this dialogue, there are many aspects a provider might reflect, such as the student's statement that things can get out of hand or the statement about the need to decide ahead of time to set a limit. With more time, the provider could revisit these statements. The example above, however, shows how a conversation can proceed in a very brief time.

IMPORTANCE AND CONFIDENCE RULERS

The "Importance Ruler and Confidence Rulers" are a quick strategy for exploring importance and potentially building confidence. This technique takes approximately 10 minutes and can be extremely valuable in moderate-length interactions—when there is more time than is necessary simply to provide advice, but not enough time to conduct a full motivational interview.

When Rollnick (1998) asked smokers about their reasons for wanting to quit, their responses tended to be divided into either the personal *value* of change (e.g., its importance to them) or their perceived *ability* to change. In order for people to attempt change, they need to believe that it is important for them and *that they can do it*. We used this model in our discussion of motivation in Chapter 3. A simple way to measure importance and confidence is to ask two scaled questions:

- *On a scale of 1–10, how important is it for you to make a change in your drinking?*
- *On a scale of 1–10, how confident are you that you could make a change if you wanted to?*

After the student responds:

1. Reflect the response (e.g., "It's pretty important to you.").
2. Ask for elaboration (e.g., "What things make it important?").
3. Ask about placement on the scale:
   Why the student didn't give a lower number ("How come a 5 and not a 1?").
   What it would take to raise the student's estimate ("What would it take to raise that estimate up to, say, a 6 or 7?").

Figures 5.1 and 5.2 illustrate the rulers, and Appendix F reproduces both of the rulers on a single page. Below each are examples of responses students might give—low, medium, and high estimates—as well as dialogue that might be appropriate given these different answers. While questions can be asked about the scales in both directions, some subtlety can be helpful. In particular, we ask about reasons it *is* important ("Why not lower?"), as opposed to reasons it's *not* important ("Why not higher?"). Likewise, we focus on reflecting reasons the student *is* confident, and ways he or she could become *more* confident. The answers to both these questions are change talk.

On a scale of 1–10, how important is it for you to make a change in your drinking?

| 1 | 2 | 3 | 4 | 5 | 6 | 7 | 8 | 9 | 10 |

Not at all important   Extremely important

Low estimate	Medium estimate	High estimate
Student: A 1.	**Student: I don't know . . . I guess about a 3.**	**Student: Probably a 9 or so.**
Counselor: Okay, so it's not that important to you at this time. I wonder if I can provide you with a little information about . . ."	Counselor: So, about in the lower middle. But I'm wondering, why did you say a 3 and not a 1? So, one reason it's important is . . . What else . . . ?	Counselor: So it's very important for you to do something about your drinking. Why is that? So, one reason it's important is . . . What else . . . ?

FIGURE 5.1. Importance Ruler. Adapted from Miller and Rollnick (2002). Copyright 2002 by The Guilford Press. Adapted by permission.

On a scale of 1–10, how confident are you that you could make a change if you wanted to?

| 1 | 2 | 3 | 4 | 5 | 6 | 7 | 8 | 9 | 10 |

Not at all confident   Extremely confident

Low estimate	Medium estimate	High estimate
Student: A one.	**Student: I don't know . . .** **I guess about a 4.**	**Student: A 10.**
Counselor: Hmm . . . Pretty low. What would it take to raise that 1 up to, say, a 5? Tell me about a change you made in the past. How did you go about it?	Counselor: So, about in the middle. But why a 4 and not a 1? What else . . . ? What would it take to raise your confidence to, say, an 8? How would you go about it? How can I be of help?	Counselor: So, you're quite confident. How would you go about it? What would it look like? What else . . . ? How would you go about it? How can I be of help?

FIGURE 5.2. Confidence Ruler. Adapted from Miller and Rollnick (2002). Copyright 2002 by The Guilford Press. Adapted by permission.

It is important not to rush the student along in the discussion of importance. Ask the student what other reasons he or she might have (e.g., "What else?"). Pause, and wait for an answer. Most students can identify at least three or four reasons.

The Confidence Ruler can also be a springboard to help students develop a plan of action. Identifying specific goals, writing the plan down, and scheduling a follow-up session can be helpful in solidifying change efforts. Below is a dialogue that might occur during a brief interaction. In this scenario, a female student is being seen in the emergency room because of an ankle sprained while drinking.

COUNSELOR: So tell me this, on a scale of 1–10, how important is it for you to make a change in your drinking? *[open-ended question]*

STUDENT: I guess about a 5.

COUNSELOR: So, about in the middle range. *[reflection]*

STUDENT: Yeah, I would say 0, but I'm a little freaked out that I hurt myself.

COUNSELOR: It makes sense that you would be concerned. What things make it important? Why a 5 and not a 1? *[reflection, open-ended question]*

STUDENT: Well, it would be nice not to have this happen again!

COUNSELOR: That would be nice! What else? *[affirmation, open-ended question]*

This student is in the middle range of importance. She has indicated that there are important reasons for her to cut down. In response, the interviewer probes to find out what these reasons are. The dialogue is similar for the confidence question below. Since the student gives a low estimate, the interviewer asks what it would take to boost her confidence. When the student mentions that she could spend more time with church friends, the interviewer helps the student arrive at a more concrete plan.

> COUNSELOR: Using the same scale, how confident are you that you could cut down or quit, if you wanted to? *[open-ended question]*
>
> STUDENT: Not that confident. Maybe a 2.
>
> COUNSELOR: Hmm . . . a little low. But why not a 1? *[reflection, open-ended question]*
>
> STUDENT: Well, I'm not addicted or anything. It would just be hard when all my friends drink.
>
> COUNSELOR: What would it take to get your confidence up a little higher, say, a 5 or even a 7 or 8? *[open-ended question]*
>
> STUDENT: Well, I would definitely have to find some people who aren't drinkers to hang around with. I guess I could start hanging out with people from my church. They don't drink.
>
> COUNSELOR: That's a good idea. What would that look like? How would you go about that? *[affirmation, open-ended question]*
>
> STUDENT: I guess I could go to church this Sunday.

CLOSING THE INTERACTION

In closing the brief interaction, we recommend a short summary, an affirmation of the student's desires or plans to change, and affirmations of statements that support self-efficacy. A follow-up visit or referral to other services may also be appropriate:

- *Thanks for talking with me. It seems to you that things are okay, but I do have some concerns. I'd like to talk to you a little more when we have time. Would that be all right?*
- *I'm impressed with the way you've thought this through. I'd like to call you in a week and follow up. What's a good time to call?*
- *Thanks for agreeing to think about this. The fall you took at the last party was a scare, and I do think that you would benefit by trying some of the strategies we talked about. I appreciate you talking to me.*
- *Maybe this isn't the right time for you. I just wanted you to know that I am here if you need to talk about this. It can stay just between the two of us.*

Finally, it is critical to close the interaction on a positive note, no matter what the student has decided. In most cases, we are merely planting the seed for change and want to leave the door open to further interactions. *Always end on good terms!*

- *Thanks for talking to me today. I appreciate you coming in.*
- *You came up with a number of really good ideas.*
- *I think your plans to . . . will really help you out.*

In the next two sections, we provide two examples of brief interventions. In the first section, we outline a 3- to 10-minute intervention that utilizes brief screening, advice, and referral. In the second section, a slightly longer time (10–30 minutes) allows for more assessment questions, the importance–confidence activity, and negotiating a plan for change. This second model, the behavioral consultation, makes more strategic uses of questions and reflections to draw out change talk.

SAMPLE BRIEF ADVICE (3–10 MINUTES)

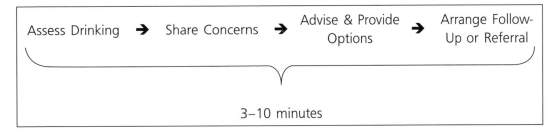

1. Using quantity–frequency questions, briefly assess the student's drinking (see Chapter 3). If possible, ask the student to complete the AUDIT prior to the meeting. Alternatively, ask the student the first three questions from the AUDIT (below). Reflect or summarize the student's responses.
   a. *How often do you have a drink containing alcohol?*
   b. *How many drinks containing alcohol do you have on a typical day when you are drinking?*
   c. *How often do you have six drinks or more on one occasion?*

2. If the student reports heavy drinking or significant drinking-related problems, share your concerns or ask the student for his or her own concerns. Use the E-P-E format to provide advice or information.
   a. *What concerns do you have about your alcohol use?*
   b. *As your doctor/counselor, I am concerned about how alcohol is affecting your . . . This accident is a direct result of your . . .*
   c. *What do you think you'd like to do about this?*

3. If appropriate, negotiate a plan of action and/or provide a menu of options. Emphasize the student's personal choice over his or her course of action.

  a. *How do you think you might be able to go about . . . ?*
  b. *Some students have found. . . . Which of these do you think will work for you?*
  c. *Ultimately, you're the one who will have to make a choice as to what you'd like to do about this.*

4. Arrange a follow-up meeting or referral. Indicate that you (or others) are available to provide assistance and support.
  a. *I'd like to schedule another appointment for about 2 weeks from now, so I can see how you're doing. I'd also like to call you (or have one of my staff call you) in a couple of days to check in with you. What's a good time to reach you?*
  b. *I'm going to give you some information that I'd like you to look over before we meet again. Would that be all right?*

5. Contact (or have someone else contact) the student within 1–2 days. A further evaluation can be arranged at this time, or a brief assessment can be administered over the phone, and the student can be mailed feedback (see, Chapter 6, "Drinking Feedback" section, p. 86). During subsequent interactions, review the student's progress and affirm efforts to cut down or abstain.

SAMPLE BEHAVIORAL CONSULTATION (10–30 MINUTES)

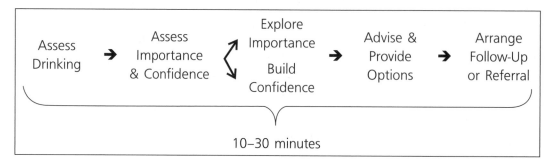

1. If possible, have the student complete the AUDIT prior to the meeting. Begin the interaction with an open-ended question about alcohol use. Follow up with either the weekly calendar questions (see Chapter 3) or the first three questions from the AUDIT. If more time is available, ask about the "Good Things, Not-So-Good Things About Drinking" (see Chapter 6). Reflect or summarize the student's responses.
  a. *Tell me a little bit about your drinking.*
  b. *About how many times per week do you have something to drink?*
  c. *When you drink, about how many drinks do you consume in a typical day?*
  d. *During the last month, what's the most you consumed on one occasion?*

e. [If time] *In your experience, what have been some of the good things about alcohol? What have been some of the not-so-good things?*

If the student reports heavy drinking or significant drinking-related consequences, ask the importance–confidence questions and follow up based on the student's response (see section on Importance and Confidence Rulers, p. 67). (The questions can be worded, as below, in terms of how important it is to *change* or in terms of risk management, e.g., "How important is it for you not to drink more than about three to four drinks in one night?" or "How important is it for you to be safe when you're drinking?").

a. *On a scale of 1–10, how important is it for you to make a change?*

b. *On a scale of 1–10, how confident are you that you could change if you wanted to?*

2. If the student indicates some interest in change, ask, "What things will be helpful to you in drinking more moderately (or safely)?" If the student shows less interest in changing, ask about change in the hypothetical: "If you wanted to drink more moderately (or safely), how would you go about it? What would you do?" If appropriate, use the E-P-E format to advise the student and/or provide a menu of options (see section on Providing Advice and Suggestions, page 63). Emphasize the student's personal choice over his or her course of action.

3. Arrange a follow-up meeting or referral. Indicate that you (or others) are available to provide assistance and support.

a. *I'd like to schedule another appointment for about 2 weeks from now, so I can see how you're doing. I'd also like to call you (or have one of my staff call you) in a couple of days to check in with you. What's a good time to reach you?*

b. *I'm going to give you some information that I'd like you to look over before we meet again. Would that be all right?*

4. Contact (or have someone else contact) the student within 1–2 days. A further evaluation can be arranged at this time, or a brief assessment can be administered over the phone, and the student can be mailed feedback (see Chapter 6, "Drinking Feedback" section). During subsequent interactions, support efforts to cut down or abstain, affirm the student for making changes, and offer additional support.

KEY POINTS

- *Brief interactions can impact high-risk drinking and reinforce safe practices.* Although different in format, brief advice and behavioral consultation share many stylistic elements with longer interventions.

- Do not assume that the student shares your concerns about alcohol or will immediately respond to a message of moderation or abstinence. Also, do not assume that every college drinker *needs* to change.
- In broaching the subject, *share your concerns* and *ask the student about his or her own concerns.*
- *Ask for permission* before giving advice, and preface advice with permission to disagree/disregard.
- When making suggestions, *be clear and specific. Provide several options* and ask the student which one will work for him or her.
- Use the elicit–provide–elicit format to provide advice or information.
- For reluctant students, *talk about change in the hypothetical.* Ask about thoughts, opinions, and plans without assuming that the student already wants to change.
- *Ask scaled questions* (e.g., "On a scale of 1–10 . . .") about the importance and confidence of change. Ask why the student is not at a lower number and what it would take to get him or her to a higher number.
- *End the interaction on a positive note.* Leave the door open to further conversations.

6

Extended Individual Interactions

OVERVIEW OF THE CHAPTER

Opportunities to talk with college students about alcohol come in all shapes and sizes. In this chapter, we discuss an intervention that is appropriate when more than just a brief time is available—what we call a *motivational* intervention. These opportunities can vary from one 45-minute meeting to several hour-long sessions. In contrast to the brief interactions described in Chapter 5, we now have greater latitude for using MI techniques. For instance, though brief advice or behavioral consultation might employ questions and reflections to encourage the student to talk about alcohol, the motivational intervention employs *particular* questions and *selective* reflections designed to diffuse resistance and increase motivation.

In our opinion, the motivational intervention is the gold standard for interacting with students about alcohol. Because of the greater length and more sophisticated delivery, a motivational intervention is likely to be appropriate when students have self-referred or have been mandated to counseling for alcohol-related difficulties. As reviewed in Chapter 2, this model of intervention has been evaluated in several controlled studies (Baer, Kivlahan, Blume, McKnight, & Marlatt, 2001; Borsari & Carey, 2000; Larimer et al., 2001; Marlatt et al., 1998; Murphy et al., 2001). Detailed protocols include the BASICS manual (Dimeff et al., 1999) and a report from the NIAAA Task Force on College Drinking (Flemming, 2002).[1]

In this chapter, we describe some general methods for beginning and ending sessions, as well as transitioning between sessions. We then present a series of MI-based exercises that are designed to facilitate contemplation and elicit change talk. Finally, we give an example of one multisession counseling protocol.

---

[1]Available at www.collegedrinkingprevention.gov/reports.

In addition to the material we provide in this chapter, extended sessions may also allow counselors the time to provide some basic information about alcohol. Although we tend to assume that young people know how alcohol works, many college students are indeed uninformed or misinformed. Topics such as the alcohol content of common drinks, absorption and metabolism of alcohol, tolerance, and the biphasic response can all be addressed. Basic alcohol-related information is available through books such as the BASICS manual (Dimeff et al., 1999) and many public websites.[2] The Alcohol "Pop Quiz" (discussed in Chapter 7 and provided in Appendix K) provides one method for introducing information. However, in providing information, we caution the counselor to ask permission first and always maintain a supportive and respectful stance. An overemphasis on giving information can lose the benefits of MI. If at all possible, elicit what the student *does* know and what concerns he or she has about alcohol. A two-way conversation is almost always better than a lecture.

OPENING AND CLOSING LONGER INTERACTIONS

The first few minutes of an interaction are critical. The counselor must establish rapport, set an agenda, and prime the student to begin talking about alcohol. Likewise, the last few minutes are also important. The counselor attempts to end the session on good terms (no matter what!) and, if appropriate, agree on a specific plan for change. For these reasons, we start this chapter by discussing the opening and closing sections of an extended interaction.

The First Few Minutes

First, *assume the student will be defensive.* Consider the context of the interview. Most students will not attend simply based on interest. Because the flavor of the early interaction will set the stage for what comes later, the spirit you convey is critical. The best questions and comments are those that show you are honestly interested in the student's point of view. If a student feels that his or her comments will be used to judge, condemn, belittle, or otherwise criticize, the spirit of the interaction will turn sour.

Next, *thank the student* for being there (even if he or she has little choice). Then *acknowledge potential awkwardness or resistance* to being there. Finally, *provide structure* so the student knows what to expect. Be clear about confidentiality and your reporting role, if any. Also explain if there are limits to confidentiality, such as in the case of suicidality or child abuse. Here's an example:

> COUNSELOR: Hi. My name is _____. I really appreciate you coming in. *[introduction, affirmation]*
>
> STUDENT: Well, they said I had to come or get booted from the dorm.

---

[2]For more information, see www.collegedrinkingprevention.gov, www.factsontap.org, or www.jointogether.org.

COUNSELOR: Yeah, I know how that happens. Still, it's great that you came in anyway. It must be a bit uncomfortable for you to be told what to do and to be expected to talk about alcohol with a counselor. *[affirmation, reflection]*

STUDENT: Yeah, not my choice of what to do today! But it ain't so bad.

COUNSELOR: Great. Let me tell you what to expect. I'll begin by asking a few questions and trying to get to know you a bit. I'll also ask you to fill out some forms, so that we can give you some feedback about what we learn. . . . It's important that you know that everything that is said here is completely confidential—I can't talk to your parents or anyone else about what you say. I do need to report to residence life that you came in, but I don't include anything about what was said. *[explanation]*

Next, ask an *open-ended* question about the student's alcohol use and *reflect* the response immediately. For instance:

- *Tell me a little bit about your drinking.*
- *Help me understand a little about how you drink.*
- *From your perspective, what happened to bring you here?* (This is especially good for students mandated to complete an alcohol program.)

Here's an example. The frequency of reflections shows that the counselor is listening:

COUNSELOR: Tell me a little bit about your drinking. *[open-ended question]*

STUDENT: I don't drink that much, mainly just on the weekend.

COUNSELOR: Mostly on the weekend. *[reflection]*

STUDENT: Yeah, when I get together with friends.

COUNSELOR: So mostly with friends on the weekend. It's mainly a social thing. What about during the week? *[reflection, open-ended question]*

STUDENT: Maybe once or twice.

COUNSELOR: Okay, so on the weekend and a couple of times during the week. When you do drink on the weekend, about how many drinks do you have? *[reflection, request for elaboration]*

Other questions in this initial section might include:

- *What are some things you like about your drinking? What are some things you don't like about it?* [See "Good Things, Not-So-Good Things," p. 83)
- *Tell me about a recent time when you had too much to drink.*
- *When are you most likely to drink? Least likely?*
- *What difficulties have you had with alcohol? How has it gotten you in trouble?*

Additional information can be helpful in understanding the student's alcohol use. If not assessed formally, it is important to explore reasons for drinking. Most students are social drinkers, and, hence, this is a theme that often comes up when discussing drinking patterns. With whom do they drink? In what situations are they most likely to drink? What benefits are important to them? For students completing the interview based on violation of rules, it can be helpful to ask what led to the referral. Ask the student how that event compares to his or her other drinking episodes. Adjudicated students often state that they drink "like everyone else, but just got caught." No matter what the student's view on the event, it is important to maintain a neutral position. It could very well be true. Other activities like feedback can test these assumptions directly.

We recommend not trying to do too much in the initial moments of a motivational session. One of the benefits of a longer interaction is that the counselor has much more latitude and flexibility—the gift of time. The key goals of the first few minutes are to establish rapport, to let the student know that he or she will not be judged or punished, and to minimize discomfort with the process. Seek opportunities to reflect and affirm, especially for students who had little choice about participating.

Closing a Session

Just as rapport is critical in beginning a session, it is also critical at the end of one. Here are a few tips. First, *offer a summary*. You might summarize the entire session, including the student's concerns, potential difficulties, or strategies to reduce risk, or choose one aspect to focus on. Next, *ask the student for a general comment* on the session (e.g., "I'm wondering what you think of all this.") to help clarify what he or she has drawn from the session and what (if any) plans he or she has decided on. Here is an example of a student who has remained more precontemplative:

COUNSELOR: We've come almost to the end of our session, so let me summarize a bit. We talked about a number of things. It seems your drinking is pretty variable, sometimes less and sometimes pretty high. You also mentioned that you need a 3.0 to keep your scholarship, but only have a 2.8 currently, and you think that the Sunday night parties definitely contribute to that. Still, it's hard for you to think of reasons why you might need to change when you see lots of other students who drink like you. Seems like the norm. You're pretty confident you could change if you decided to. I'm wondering, what do you make of all this? *[summary, open-ended question]*

STUDENT: I still don't think it's such a big deal. Yeah, I drink . . . but there are a lot of other students who drink the way I do and don't get caught.

COUNSELOR: Sounds like you've got a lot to think about. *[reflection]*

STUDENT: Yeah.

In this example, the counselor cannot pursue a plan of action, so instead (and this is common) he or she encourages the student to think about or consider what they have discussed.

Here is an example of a (probably less typical) student who has decided to make a change over the course of the session:

> COUNSELOR: We've come almost to the end of our session, and we've talked about many things—your drinking, your concerns about your grades, prior efforts to make changes. I'm wondering, what do you make of all this? *[summary, open-ended question]*
>
> STUDENT: I don't know . . . it just seems like I've got to do something about my drinking.
>
> COUNSELOR: You think it might be good for you to make a change. *[reflection]*
>
> STUDENT: Yeah, I just never thought of myself as an "extreme" drinker. I figured that I drank about as much as everyone else. But it's really hurting my grades, and I can't afford to lose my scholarship.
>
> COUNSELOR: So, where does this leave you? *[open-ended question]*
>
> STUDENT: I just won't drink anymore. I've made up my mind.
>
> COUNSELOR: How would you do that? *[open-ended question]*

It is always appropriate to provide the student with referral information, a list of contacts, or a map to campus facilities should he or she want further assistance. In closing the session, we suggest reminding the student of any future sessions and thanking the student for speaking with you.

Despite our efforts, many students with clear difficulties will leave the interaction as precontemplators or contemplators. If you are in college counseling for the clear statements of affirmation, prepare to be disappointed! Only a minority of students will thank the interviewer or make reinforcing statements like, "Wow, I've never thought of that!" or "I've got to do something about my drinking." Students may make some change in the future, but at this point, we may simply be raising awareness and moving a student along the stages of change. In fact, when successful changers are followed up, they rarely attribute changes to the counseling interaction. This is one of the best aspects of the motivational interview. Because we encourage students to voice their own reasons and plans for change, we rarely foster dependence. Students feel empowered to make changes on their own.

In the closing moments of the session, the *most critical* goal is to leave the student with a positive experience in talking with an adult about alcohol—the experience of being listened to, cared about, not judged, not told what to do—in essence, treated as an adult. This perception allows a student to save face in the interaction—that is, it gives a student permission to think about the issues that have been discussed, without feeling that he or she has to strongly defend his or her current actions. Ending on a positive note also makes it more likely that a student will seek out additional services at some point in the future. Therefore, the goal for the last few moments of an interaction is to affirm students with statements of understanding and an acknowledgment of personal choice. *Always end on good terms*!

- *Thanks for talking to me today. I appreciate you coming in.*
- *I hope this was helpful. Of course, it's totally up to you to decide what might come next.*
- *I appreciate you talking to me. You came up with a number of really good ideas.*
- *I liked what you had to say about. . . . I really think that will work for you.*
- *I think your plans to . . . will really help you out.*

TALKING ABOUT CHANGE (WHEN IT MAKES SENSE TO DO SO)

For students who already drink moderately, the session can be focused on reinforcing current patterns or helping them with other concerns. However, for students who are having difficulties, we hope that at some point they will begin to show signs of readiness, and we can shift to a practical discussion about change. There are no hard and fast rules to determine when this should happen. Some students may begin voicing dissatisfaction with current patterns or ask for help implementing new ones. Other students may exhibit subtle shifts in language, such as:

- Less arguing, disagreeing, or negativity
- Asking fewer questions
- Changing from conditional (e.g., "may, might, can") to performative statements (e.g., "will")
- Talking about what change would be like

Although we sometimes see these overt behaviors, in our experience, it is only the minority of students who will show clear interest in change. Students who "see the light" during treatment sessions are relatively rare. Rather, we recognize that, for most students, we are merely planting the seed for change or, better yet, encouraging them to think about drinking in a different way so as to make change more attractive or likely in the future.

If the counselor is unsure whether to proceed, it may be helpful to test the waters with a transitional question like:

- *What are you thinking you'd like to do about this?*
- *Where does this leave you in terms of your drinking?*

While suggestions and advice from a counselor can sometimes be helpful, it is generally better for the student to arrive at his or her own plan. Thus, we do everything we can to draw out solutions and plans from the student. If the student appears motivated but seems to have genuine difficulty identifying ways to reduce harm, it can be appropriate to provide him or her with a menu of options (see Chapter 5). Two worksheets found in the Appendices ("Goal Setting," Appendix N and "Strategies for Low-Risk Drinking," Appendix M) can also help structure students' ideas about change. As we mentioned in Chapter 5, in providing advice, it is important to *ask permission* and to *leave the onus for change with the student*.

Here's an example:

COUNSELOR: Well, thanks for sticking in there. I know that feedback information was a little difficult to take, especially that stuff on family history of alcoholism. But I'm wondering, where does all of this leave you in terms of your drinking? *[affirmation, open-ended question]*

STUDENT: Well, if I could I would quit right now. I'm tempted to, but it would be really weird with my friends.

COUNSELOR: So quitting might be difficult for you. *[reflection]*

STUDENT: I just wish there were some other way. I mean, do you think it's possible for someone like me to drink but not become an alcoholic?

COUNSELOR: I'm sorry to say I don't know the answer to that question. But it seems like you want to do something about it. *[reflection]*

STUDENT: Hmm . . . There is just no good way to handle this. I mean, I would feel strange around my friends if I quit drinking completely.

COUNSELOR: Would it be all right if I suggested something? *[asks for permission]*

STUDENT: Sure.

COUNSELOR: There are many ways to reduce risks. Some students find it easier to quit drinking entirely, while others have found that a trial period of moderate drinking can help them determine if it's possible for them to drink in a controlled way. *[gives advice]*

STUDENT: What do you mean?

COUNSELOR: Well, if you were interested, I wonder if we could come up with some drinking limits that make sense for you, like how much you'll drink or how often. Since we meet again in 2 weeks, you could try it out and we could discuss it the next time we meet. *[explanation]*

In this example, the counselor suggests a period of moderate drinking with a student who seems to be stuck. Depending on the student, it might be appropriate to suggest a trial period of not drinking as part of a menu of options. However, for most students, our advice will be centered on risk reduction. If a student chooses to drink, he or she should do so as safely as possible.

As we have already noted, the pattern for risky college drinking seems to be the heavy episode. Because of this, we would rather have the student reduce the number of drinks per drinking day or reduce the frequency of heavy-drinking episodes rather than reduce his or her drinking by saving up for one heavy-drinking episode. (For instance, a reduction from 1 drink per day, or 7 drinks per week, to 5 drinks per Saturday would probably not reduce the student's risk.) There are several benchmarks that students can use to select a drinking goal:

- No drinking at all
- No drinking in high-risk situations
- A maximum *number of drinks per hour* that the student will not exceed
- A maximum *number of drinks per episode* that the student will not exceed
- A maximum *BAC level* that the student will not exceed

In this planning portion of the interaction, we strongly advise counselors against pushing students to make a choice. Such a premature focus on change can have the unintended consequence of making students commit to the easiest and least complicated option available to them—maintaining the status quo. Similarly, we caution against giving simple solutions or advice that are likely to leave students more frustrated about their real world problem.

As noted in Chapter 5, if you do provide direct advice, we suggest following with a menu of options and a comment that points out the student's ultimate responsibility for change.

- *What would you like to do about it?*
- *Some students have found it helpful to . . . Which of those do you think might work for you?*
- *So, I've given you a few suggestions, but ultimately you're the one who has to make it work.*

Of course, the student's goal may be different from the counselor's. While abstinence may seem like the clearest alternative to the counselor, many students would rather try a period of moderate, controlled, or less risky drinking. Whatever the counselor's personal beliefs, it is important that he or she support the student in these chosen efforts to reduce risk and not try to *make* the student do anything.

This portion of the interaction might involve discussion of specific strategies to moderate drinking, such as: (1) identifying what the student wants from drinking, (2) choosing appropriate drinking limits, (3) identifying high-risk situations, (4) practicing drinking-refusal skills, and (5) monitoring consumption when choosing to drink. For example, to help the student arrive at a plan for change, the counselor might ask about the difficulties the student thinks he or she might encounter, such as high-risk environments (e.g., a fraternity or sorority party), internal states (e.g., anger, boredom), or relationships (e.g., wanting to meet women at a party). If the student responds well in such a situation, he or she will generally feel more confident the next time the situation occurs. On the other hand, if the student is unable to stick to his or her goals, he or she may be left with a sense of powerlessness. Most times, "slips" are less risky in and of themselves and more risky because they demoralize the student and lower his or her inhibitions to further drinking. Thus, in addition to helping the student select appropriate drinking goals, the counselor may also mention that a slip does not mean that the student needs to give up on efforts to do things differently.

MOTIVATIONAL EXERCISES

There are many options available for those conducting longer individual sessions. On one end, one can proceed with little structure, using the MI techniques discussed in Chapter 4 to explore feelings about alcohol and the possibility of change. However, many students do not easily engage in these conversations, and sometimes conversations take side trips into other areas. Fortunately, MI practitioners have developed a number of relatively simple exercises that can structure and facilitate the process. The exercises below are designed to encourage discussion of pros and cons of drinking, highlight patterns of use, and explore and understand reasons for drinking. These exercises can be a great help—they provide a structured way to keep the conversation on track.

Good Things, Not-So-Good Things (5–10 Minutes)

People drink for many different reasons, and often see some real benefits from even the most problematic behaviors. The "Good Things, Not-So-Good Things" activity—often used near the beginning of an interaction—helps students explore ambivalence about drinking. The exercise can be conducted in two ways. One way is to ask the student to generate two lists related to current *drinking*: "Good Things about Drinking" and "Not-So-Good Things about Drinking." The other way is to ask students to make two lists related to *change*: "Reasons for Change" and "Reasons for Staying the Same."

In this example, the counselor asks the student to identify pros and cons of drinking. Although it is possible to do this activity without actually writing out the student's responses, this counselor keeps two lists, "Good Things" and "Not-So-Good Things." The counselor starts out asking about the "Good Things," reflects the student's responses, and asks for the "Not-So-Good" things. The counselor then asks for the "Not-So-Good" things. Figure 6.1 shows what the resulting list might look like.

COUNSELOR: So let me see if I have this right. You drink mostly on the weekends, but occasionally during the week if it's not basketball season. You told me you drink

Good things about drinking	Not-so-good things about drinking
Social interaction	Throwing up, hangovers
Get along with friends	Makes me fatter
Helps me relax	Costs money
Quenches thirst	Girlfriend nags me
Relieves pain	Periods of blackout
Like taste	RA lectures me

FIGURE 6.1. Sample "Good Things, Not-So-Good Things" list.

with friends on the weekend, but mostly alone during the week. You estimated that you might have 5–10 beers on a weekend night and maybe 2–3 during a weeknight. Have I got that right? *[summarization]*

STUDENT: Yeah, that's about right. Except that it's more like 5 beers on a weekend night. Ten beers would be really pushing it.

COUNSELOR: Okay, thanks for clarifying that. Would it be all right if we did a short exercise? Let me ask you this: What are some things you like about your drinking? *[asks for permission, open-ended question]*

STUDENT: I don't know . . . I guess it's fun when you're with friends.

COUNSELOR: So maybe to get along with others or to liven things up. Okay, let me write that down. What else? *[reflection, open-ended question]*

STUDENT: Well, I guess it helps me to relax . . .

COUNSELOR: Okay, let's try the other side. What are some of the not-so-good things about drinking? *[open-ended question]*

STUDENT: Hangovers! Puking. Weight gain . . .

In generating these lists, the student has illustrated the classic dilemma: feeling two ways about something. A summary and double-sided reflection capture this nicely.

COUNSELOR: So it seems like alcohol, for you, is a mixed bag. On the one hand, your drinking helps you to fit in with friends and relax after a hard day at school. But on the other hand, you can sometimes end up drinking more than you wanted to. *[summarization]*

STUDENT: Well, yeah. Plus, it really bothers my girlfriend. I mean, she's not against drinking or anything, but I can come off as an ass when I've been drinking. It's just tough . . .

COUNSELOR: Sort of tough not knowing what to do. *[reflection]*

Just as there are pros and cons to a behavior, there are also pros and cons to *changing* a behavior. For this version, follow the above procedures in making two lists, "Reasons to Change" and "Reasons to Stay the Same." If the student gives a "Reasons to Change" list that is longer than the list of "Reasons to Stay the Same," you might point this out. You might also ask the student to assign a point value of 1–5 to each item based on how important it is. The student then totals the two lists to get a sense of which course of action is most indicated.

> COUNSELOR: Let me see if I can summarize. On the one hand, you enjoy drinking because it helps to loosen things up a bit and makes you more relaxed. You're afraid that you might lose friends if you quit and wouldn't know what to do with yourself if you weren't drinking. On the other hand, you've identified quite a few reasons for quitting. Over the past month, you've been feeling more swamped by school, and being hung over in the morning definitely doesn't help. Your girlfriend and at least one other person are concerned that your drinking is getting more out of control. By quitting, you think you also might see some health benefits, like feeling better physically and looking more attractive. Have I got that right? *[summarization]*
>
> STUDENT: Yeah, that sounds about right.
>
> COUNSELOR: You're stuck in the middle. *[reflection]*

We have sometimes encountered providers who are reluctant to use this activity because they are afraid that allowing students to talk about the benefits of drinking will *validate* the students' behavior. It is important to understand that we are not condoning the student's drinking, but merely recognizing that the student experiences some real benefits from it. An exercise like this helps set the stage for change talk, because it (1) Conveys respect for students by recognizing that their behavior has some valid purposes; (2) Gets reluctant students talking about drinking and makes it more likely that they will honestly discuss some of the negatives; (3) Identifies potential barriers to change, and; (4) Helps students visualize the pros and cons of a behavior so that they can make a more informed decision about whether they would like to make a change.

This exercise does not necessarily lead to change talk. However, after exploring both positive and negative aspects of drinking, the interviewer can reflect ambivalence and ask key questions. Some summative open-ended questions to use with this exercise include:

- *When you list it all this way, what do you think?*
- *How does this all add up?*
- *Any ideas about how you might alter the balance? More good things, fewer not-so-good things?*
- *If you chose not to drink, what are some ways you could still get these benefits?*

Drinking Feedback (20–40 Minutes)

There is good evidence that feedback presented by an empathic counselor can be effective at reducing drinking among college students (Baer et al., 1992, 2001; Borsari & Carey, 2000; Larimer et al., 2001; Marlatt et al., 1998; Murphy et al., 2001). In some cases, even mailed or web-based feedback has led to substantial drinking reductions (Agostinelli, Brown, & Miller, 1995; Collins, Carey, & Sliwinski, 2002; Neighbors, Larimer, & Lewis, 2004; Walters, 2000; Walters, Bennett, & Miller, 2000; Walters & Neighbors, 2005). Most in-person feedback interventions are structured along the lines of a health appraisal: Students complete an assessment and then meet with a counselor who presents the results. The BASICS approach (Dimeff et al., 1999) is an example of a two-session feedback intervention. Feedback consists of items that are thought to be particularly motivating to college drinkers, such as

- Quantity/frequency of drinking, peak BAC
- Comparison of the student's drinking to national or local college drinking norms
- Amount of money and percentage of income spent on alcohol
- Tolerance level, genetic risk of alcoholism
- AUDIT, RAPI, or other consequence measure
- Risky behaviors engaged in because of alcohol use
- Expectations about alcohol consumption
- Perception of drinking compared to actual amounts
- Explanation, advice, referral information

With paper feedback such as the Check-Up to Go (CHUG; Appendix G) you are limited to feedback that can be calculated by hand. In more recent years, computer-generated feedback has offered a more sophisticated look at student drinking, for instance giving feedback on calories consumed (www.e-chug.com), giving students the option to compare their drinking to specific subgroups (e.g., freshmen, Greek-affiliated, athletes; www.mystudentbody.com), or providing personalized fact sheets based on student information (www.alcoholedu.com). If you do not have access to one of these websites, you can use the CHUG assessment and feedback forms presented in Appendix G.[3] This feedback is calculated by hand and uses national college norms and referral information. Appendix G also gives background information about the CHUG and instructions for translating the assessment information onto the feedback sheet. You may wish to include local referral information in a separate insert or in the blank section at the end of the feedback.

Before conducting this exercise, the student must complete the assessment sheets (page 159), and the information must be translated onto the feedback sheets (page 162). Information from a consequence measure, such as the CAPS-r (discussed in Chapter 3, provided in Appendix C) or the YAAPST (discussed in Chapter 3, presented in Appendix

[3]An online version of the CHUG is available for a subscription fee at www.e-chug.com. A free feedback program is available at www.alcoholinnerview.com.

B), can also provide information to present as part of the feedback section. Presenting feedback involves three basic steps:

1. Give the student a copy of the feedback sheet; tell the student that he or she will be able to keep it.
2. Present each section of the feedback, moving slowly and giving background information when necessary.
3. When the student reacts to the information (verbally or nonverbally), reflect and summarize what the student is feeling.

Note what is *not* part of the three basic steps: giving advice, educating, making points, or drawing conclusions for the student. It is important to resist the natural urge to become directive when giving feedback. Let the feedback speak for itself.

Here is an example of a dialogue that starts this activity:

COUNSELOR: What I'd like to do now is give you some feedback on your drinking. The information on this feedback sheet is based on the assessments you filled out last week. It's just information for you to think about, and some students find it really helpful. Of course, any change you decide to make is totally up to you. You can take this sheet home with you. *[introduction, explanation]*

STUDENT: Okay.

COUNSELOR: This first section summarizes what you said about your drinking. Based on your information, it looks like in an average month you drink about 90 standard drinks, and that puts you at about the 95th percentile of U.S. college males in terms of your drinking. *[explanation]*

STUDENT: So what does that mean?

COUNSELOR: It means that, compared to other male U.S. college students, you drink more than about 95%, or that 5% drink more than you do. *[explanation]*

STUDENT: (*Looks surprised.*) Hmm . . .

COUNSELOR: You look a little surprised. *[reflection]*

STUDENT: Well, yeah. I'm not sure where you got your information, but that doesn't sound right.

COUNSELOR: It's hard to believe. *[reflection]*

In this example, the counselor has let the student know what to expect and presented the first item. The student reacts to the item, and the counselor reflects the student's reaction. The feedback information, rather than the counselor, is the primary motivator. It is not necessary for the student to "believe" the feedback is correct. In many cases, students will remain outwardly skeptical, while being inwardly persuaded (or at least contemplative).

Here's an example of a student being presented with feedback about negative consequences attributable to alcohol:

COUNSELOR: This next section summarizes some of the difficulties you've had as a result of your drinking. For instance, you mentioned that alcohol had caused you to miss class twice in the last month. *[explanation]*

STUDENT: It was no big deal.

COUNSELOR: It didn't seem like a big deal to you. *[reflection, open-ended question]*

STUDENT: Nah, not really.

COUNSELOR: What happened? *[open-ended question]*

STUDENT: Not much. I have this Monday class at 8:00 A.M. I guess there were a couple times that I just didn't get out of bed and slept right through. But it's okay.

COUNSELOR: So you drank a little too much and it was hard for you to get up in the morning. Okay. *(pause)* Tell me about this item here where you said that you had driven shortly after drinking. *[reflection, asks for elaboration]*

STUDENT: Well, I know it wasn't the smartest thing to do, but it was only a short way home.

COUNSELOR: So it worked out okay, but you have a sense that it wasn't exactly the safest thing to do. *[reflection]*

STUDENT: Yeah, I probably shouldn't have done that . . .

Despite the student's minimization, the counselor asks for elaboration on the concerns the student *does* have. Because the feedback is powerful, it can be tempting to confront the student with further information in an attempt to persuade him or her directly. However, *feedback is most powerful when it speaks for itself*, and the counselor is merely a guide. Resist the urge to push the student or argue about survey results, study design, calculations, etc. Affirm and reflect responses just as during other parts of the session.

- *What do you think?*
- *What do you make of that?*
- *You're surprised!*
- *Thanks for sticking with this.*

As the exercise ends, summarize the feedback information and the student's responses and ask a summative question: "What do you make of all this?"

New Roads Functional Analysis (10–15 Minutes)

The "New Roads" activity (Miller & Pechacek, 1987) is a simple exercise to help students identify why they might be drinking. We have already mentioned the Comprehensive

Effects of Alcohol measure (discussed in Chapter 3, and provided in Appendix E) as one way to gather information about alcohol expectancies. Another way is to ask the student directly what things he or she expects from alcohol and, based on that information, to imagine how they might get those effects if they chose not to drink. This activity, which typically occurs later in an interaction, is often used to preface skills-building exercises.

To begin this activity, ask the student to identify situations where he or she is likely to drink.

- *When do you feel most like drinking?*
- *When is it most difficult for you not to drink?*

Record the student's answers in a column on the left side of a page under the heading, "Triggers." After the student has listed several items, create a second column, labeled "Effects," to the right of the Triggers column. Ask the student to describe several of the things he or she enjoys about drinking.

- *What things do you like about alcohol?*
- *What are some of the good things about your drinking?*

COUNSELOR: Help me understand a bit more about how you drink. Earlier you mentioned that you drink at parties. So what are you feeling before you drink? I mean, what prompted you to have a drink in the first place? *[explanation open-ended question]*

STUDENT: I guess I have a drink to loosen up.

COUNSELOR: So, maybe you're feeling a little tense or anxious, and alcohol makes you more relaxed. Let me write that down here. What else? *[reflection, open-ended question]*

STUDENT: It helps me talk to women.

COUNSELOR: What do you mean? *[request for elaboration]*

STUDENT: It can be hard to approach a girl. I'm not the most confident guy in the world.

COUNSELOR: Okay, so you'd like to be able to approach a girl you like, but you're afraid you won't know what to say. *[reflection]*

STUDENT: Yeah, it helps me not to be afraid . . . to be more confident . . . (*Counselor fills in the Triggers column.*)

COUNSELOR: Okay, that's a good list. Now how about some of the things you like about drinking? *[affirmation, open-ended question]*

STUDENT: Well, it helps me get to sleep.

COUNSELOR: Okay, sleep. I'll write that down here under the heading "Effects." What else? *[reflection, open-ended question]*

STUDENT: Well, I mentioned before that a big one for me is that I feel more confident when I've been drinking. Like it's easier to meet people.

COUNSELOR: Courage. What else? (*Continues filling in the Effects column.*) [*reflection, open-ended question*]

After completing the two columns, help the student *draw lines* from items in the Triggers column to items in the Effects column. These lines link antecedents with their consequences. Figure 6.2 gives an example of a completed list. For example, "shyness" in the Triggers column might connect with "feel more comfortable" in the Effects column. At the end, every item on each list should connect to one or more items on the other list.

COUNSELOR: Now what I'd like to do is draw a line from each item in this Triggers list to an item in the Effects list. Help me with this (*points at first item*). When you feel tense or anxious, and you have a drink, which of these things happens (*points at Effects items*)? [*open-ended question*]

STUDENT: Um . . . I guess that goes with "Feel relaxed."

COUNSELOR: Okay. How about "Afraid"? [*open-ended question*]

STUDENT: I guess it goes with "Courage."

Finally, circle the items in the Triggers column and ask the student how, if he or she chose not to drink, he or she could still get the same effects. This begins the search for alternative coping strategies. For example, if the student chose not to drink, another way to relieve tension might be to play basketball. Instead of using alcohol to quench thirst, he or she might drink water. A second chart (Figure 6.3) lists "Effects" as well as these "Alternative Strategies."

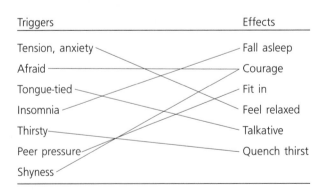

FIGURE 6.2. Sample "Triggers" and "Effects" columns. Adapted from Miller and Pechacek (1987). Copyright 1987 by Elsevier. Adapted by permission.

Effects	Jim's alternative strategies
Get to sleep	Wake up on time
Courage	Ask a friend for an introduction
Accepted by others	Just be yourself, they will accept you
Feel relaxed	Enroll in yoga class
Forget, escape	Exercise, run after class
Talkative	Exercise, run after class (endorphins!)
Quench thirst	Drink water or nonalcoholic beverage
Relieve craving	Drink only one beer and then reevaluate

FIGURE 6.3. Sample alternative strategies.

[Circles "Effects" column.] *What I'm curious about is, supposing you decided not to drink on a particular evening. How would you still get these effects? I mean, let's say you're at a party. How would you loosen up if you chose not to drink?*

As we discussed in Chapter 5, strategies are discussed in the hypothetical. That is, students are asked to come up with a list of behaviors they might do, *if they chose not to drink*. Finish the activity by providing the student with a copy of "Strategies for Low-Risk Drinking" (Appendix M) and ask him or her to complete the sheet before the next session.

Values Cardsort (15–30 Minutes)

This exercise allows students to identify those life values that are most important to them and weigh these in relation to their current patterns of drinking. This activity is useful in longer interactions.

Begin this activity by explaining that people tend to hold a core set of values that guide their behaviors. Because everyone is unique, no two people are exactly alike in their priorities. Hand the student the deck of "values" cards (Miller & C'de Baca, 2001; the cards in Appendix H are formatted to be duplicated on preperforated business card paper) and explain that these 70 cards contain potentially important life values. Flip through and point out several of the values in the deck. Ask the student to select the 10 values that are most important to him or her and prioritize this top ten from most to least important.

COUNSELOR: I'd like to do a little exercise with you that most students seem to like. (*Hands students the deck of cards.*) On each of these cards is a potentially important life value—something that people find important. I'd like you to pick out the 10 values that are the most important to you. *[instruction]* (*Student sorts the cards.*) Now, I'd like you to put those ten in order from most important to least important. *[instruction]* (*Student sorts the cards.*)

Figure 6.4 shows what a resulting list might look like. After the student has finished sorting his or her top 10, the counselor asks the student to elaborate on the items.

- *I see that you put "family" in the first spot. Why is that?*
- *People sometimes mean different things when they use the word "genuineness." What do you mean by it? Give me an example . . .*
- *How does that affect the way you act?*

Next, help the student to weigh his or her values in relation to current drinking. One way to do this is to simply ask the student how drinking fits in with his or her values. Another way is to have the student physically sort the cards in relation to his or her current drinking. For this second option, draw three circles on a blank page, and label them "+" "0" and "−" (i.e., plus, zero, and minus). Ask the student to sort the values into the three piles based on how each value relates to his or her drinking (i.e., my drinking helps me to get, has no relation to, or hinders me from getting this value). When the student is finished sorting, ask him or her to elaborate on the placement of the cards. Reflect and affirm the student's responses, particularly those that indicate discrepancy or concern.

COUNSELOR: Okay, one more thing. I've drawn three circles on this page, a plus, zero, and minus. I want you to sort your list into these three piles based on whether your drinking helps you to get that value, is unrelated, or hinders you from getting it. *[instruction]*

STUDENT: My drinking now?

COUNSELOR: Your current drinking. (*Student sorts the cards.*) So how did you sort them? *[open-ended question]*

STUDENT: Well, most of them went into the minus pile. It was hard to know where to put "friends," so I just put it in the middle.

---

1. Family—*to have a happy, loving family*
2. Friends—*to have close, supportive friends*
3. Genuineness—*to behave in a manner that is true to who I am*
4. God's will—*to seek and obey the will of God*
5. Loved—*to be loved by those close to me*
6. Loving—*to give love to others*
7. Adventure—*to have new and exciting experiences*
8. Contribution—*to make a contribution that will last after I am gone*
9. Risk—*to take risks and challenges*
10. Humor—*to see the humorous side of myself and the world*

FIGURE 6.4. Sample prioritized values.

COUNSELOR: So it looks like for most things, your current drinking is not fitting in. *[reflection]*

STUDENT: Yeah, especially the "family" thing. And the "God's will" thing.

COUNSELOR: Why is that? *[open question]*

Allow the student time to talk about the connection between values and drinking. As the exercise ends, summarize the student's responses and ask a summative question: "What do you make of all this?"

There are instances where students identify, either honestly or dishonestly, values that would seem to contraindicate moderate drinking. For instance, if a student's top values are adventure, popularity, sexuality, fun, and humor, it may be difficult to see how a reduction in drinking would help a student get *more* of these. On the contrary, some students drink heavily precisely because heavy drinking fits into their personal value system. In these instances, asking students to elaborate on the connection between values and drinking may actually reinforce the status quo. There are several natural stopping points in this exercise, and counselors will have to use their own judgment about when to wrap it up with a phrase like:

- *Sometimes it's interesting to consider how drinking fits into your broader values.*
- *As your values change over the next 5 years, I hope you'll be able to take a new look at how drinking fits into your life.*

Self-Monitoring Cards (10–20 Minutes, Two Visits)

Self-monitoring—keeping track of what, how much, and during what circumstances alcohol is consumed—is one way to raise awareness of drinking patterns. Some studies have asked students to keep track of their drinking as part of a counseling intervention (Baer et al., 1992; Larimer et al., 2001; Marlatt et al., 1998). Used in this way, a completed self-monitoring card provides information that may be useful to the counselor when providing advice or feedback. Other studies have used self-monitoring as the actual intervention (Garvin, Alcorn, & Faulkner, 1990; Nye, Agostinelli, & Smith, 1999). As we describe it below, self-monitoring involves at least two interactions—one to explain how to complete the cards and a subsequent one (or ones) to review the student's drinking diary.

During the first interaction, ask the student to keep a daily diary of his or her drinking until the next meeting. Give the student several wallet-sized self-monitoring cards (Appendix I) and explain how to complete the cards. In the column "Date," write in the dates that the card will cover (e.g., each day of the week following the session).

Instruct the student to make one entry each day, filling in the spaces to indicate how much he or she drank, over what time of day, and where he or she was when drinking. Explain that you are not asking him or her to change anything—only to keep track of what is consumed. There are spaces on the card for different kinds of alcohol (i.e., beer, wine, and liquor) that are summed for each day under the column, "Total Number of Drinks." There is also a space where the student can describe the situation in which he or she drank. *To achieve best results, the cards should be completed as close as possible to when the student is drinking.* Students may be uncomfortable with the idea of recording drinks in the middle of a party, so this needs to be discussed in a respectful way. Ask the student what difficulties the student thinks he or she might have completing the cards.

> COUNSELOR: I have one more thing I'd like to talk about. It's a little more complicated than what we've done so far, but a lot of students find it really helpful. I'd like to challenge you to keep track of your drinking from now until we meet next week. Now, I'm not asking you to make any changes, I'd just like you to keep a little diary of how much you're drinking to give us both a better picture of how you're drinking. It should just take a couple of minutes a day. Would you be willing to do this? *[instruction]*

> STUDENT: Sure, I guess. I'm not sure what good it would do.

> COUNSELOR: Okay. I'd like you to put your information on these little cards. Basically, there's one row for each day. I want you to keep track of how many drinks you had on that day—there are separate spaces for beer, wine, and liquor or mixed drinks. There is also a space where you can write in a word or two description, like if you were at a party, watching TV, or doing something else. To get an accurate number, it's important that the cards are completed every day. And you'll get the most out of this if you record your drinks *while* you are drinking, so that your impressions aren't from memory. *[instruction]*

> STUDENT: You want me to pull these out in the middle of a party?

> COUNSELOR: Well, actually, yes. I know it's a bit odd, but it will help you learn a lot about your decisions to drink. How might you manage that? Is there anything you could do or say that would make it easier? *[instruction, open-ended question]*

> STUDENT: Well, I could say it's for a class. Or (*pause*) would it be okay if I went to the bathroom or something to fill them out?

> COUNSELOR: Sure! Whatever works for you. I've had some people say they were doing an experiment. Others say they're keeping track of their diet. *[menu of options]*

> STUDENT: Would it be okay to just write down what I had after the party?

> COUNSELOR: Of course it's okay. I think you'll get more out of it if you do it at the time. But do what seems right for you. Your choice. *[emphasis on personal choice]*

> STUDENT: What if I forget to fill it out?

> COUNSELOR: Good question. If you really have difficulty filling it out at night, it's okay to do it the next day. But we find that the information is much more accurate and helpful if it is filled in as close as possible to when you drink. *[affirmation, instruction]*

Self-monitoring cards can also be used when students have identified a specific drinking goal. It is possible, for instance, for the student to pick a drinking limit for a particular day and write the number in parentheses on the card as a reminder. If there are discrepancies between the student's goal and what he or she actually consumed, the counselor and student can discuss them.

During a follow-up session, discuss the self-monitoring cards with the student. Begin this portion with an open-ended question like "How did the diary cards go?" The response to a question like this will give an idea of whether the diary is likely to be valid. For instance, if a student responds that he or she had a hard time with the task and only kept the diary sporadically, you may want to ask him or her to repeat the exercise. The counselor might also explore why it was difficult for the student to complete the cards. Next, explore the specific content of the diary, asking the student to describe how much he or she drank overall and on peak occasions. Ask the student to describe days that stand out on the diary card (e.g., heavy or abstinent days) and to identify factors that influenced his or her drinking. Finally, ask an open-ended question about what the student learned from the task, such as, "You've been watching your drinking closely for the last week. What have you noticed?" At this point, we are interested in the insights, surprises, or thoughts the student had as a result.

- *What was it like? What did you learn?*
- *In general, what times of the week do you drink the most?*
- *What things made it hard for you to stick to your drinking goal?*
- *What people had a particularly positive/negative influence on your drinking?*
- *What things would you like to do differently the next time?*

After reviewing the diary cards, ask the student if he or she would like to set a new drinking goal or adjust the current goal and encourage him or her to repeat the exercise over the next week. If time is available, you may also instruct the student how to calculate his or her BAC for one heavy episode in the diary (see Chapter 3) or give the student a personalized BAC card. Appendix J contains reproducible BAC cards for males and females. For a more personalized card, BAC Zone sells laminated BAC cards that are customized based on gender and weight.[4]

SAMPLE MOTIVATIONAL INTERVENTION (FOUR SESSIONS, 60 MINUTES EACH)

This section provides an example of how several motivational techniques and activities might be integrated into an individual intervention. This example consists of an initial assessment session and three subsequent meetings, scheduled approximately 2 weeks

---

[4]For ordering information, see www.baczone.biz.

apart. During the first session, the student is oriented to the clinical protocol, completes an assessment packet, and schedules a follow-up session. Information from the assessments is used to generate feedback for the second session. The second session, which includes a presentation of feedback, is primarily focused on helping the student explore and resolve ambivalence. The third session stresses skills techniques, and the fourth focuses on clarifying values and planning for the future. While our example spans four sessions, effective motivational interventions can be completed with just two or three sessions.

Motivational Intervention Session 1: Assessment

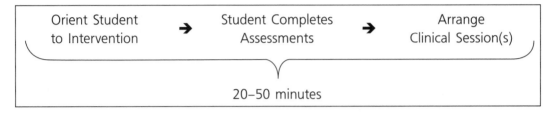

1. Orient the student to the protocol (e.g., number of sessions, meeting times, focus of sessions, reporting procedure).

2. Hand the student the assessment instruments and explain that the information he or she provides will help you to understand better where he or she is coming from. His or her responses will also be used to generate a personalized drinking profile that you will present next session. (The number and/or content of clinical sessions can also be determined by the student's assessment results.) Encourage the student to be honest in his or her responses. Chapter 3 offers suggestions for choosing specific instruments. Table 6.1 summarizes assessment batteries that might be appropriate given different time constraints. The Check-Up to Go (CHUG) is included in each instance because it includes information necessary for generating

TABLE 6.1. Recommended Assessment Packages Based on Available Time

Approximate time	Information gathered	Instrument	Page
5–10 minutes	Consumption and feedback information	CHUG Assessment	159
10–20 minutes	Consumption and feedback information	CHUG Assessment	159
	Negative consequences	CAPS-r	146
	Readiness to change	RTCQ	149
20–30 minutes	Consumption and feedback information	CHUG Assessment	159
	Negative consequences	YAAPST	140
	Readiness to change	RTCQ	149
	Drinking expectancies	CEOA	153

the personal feedback report (though another feedback protocol would also work). The AUDIT is included in the CHUG assessment sheet.

3. If there is additional time, introduce self-monitoring cards (see section on self-monitoring cards, p. 93). Give the student several cards, explain how to complete them, and tell him or her that you will review the cards together during the next session.

Motivational Intervention Session 2

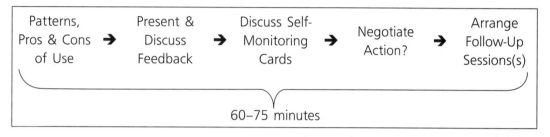

1. *Thank the student for attending* (see section on The First Few Minutes, p. 76). *Review confidentiality and other site procedures. Lay out the basic structure of the session. Thank the student for filling out the assessments during the last session and tell him or her that you will be presenting some information students often find helpful.*

2. Begin with an open-ended question about alcohol use. (Since the student has completed drinking assessments, you will presumably already have some information about the student's consumption and risk factors.) Reflect the student's responses. (See section on The First Few Minutes, p. 76.)
   a. *Tell me a little bit about your drinking.*
   b. *When are you most/least likely to drink?*
   c. *In what situations is it hardest for you not to drink?*
   d. *In your experience, what have been some of the good things about drinking? What have been some of the not-so-good things?* (See section on Good Things, Not-So-Good Things, p. 83.)

3. Using information from the BAC cards, explore the student's drinking profile, including amount drank overall, heavier episodes, and abstinent days (see section on Self-Monitoring Cards, p. 93). Explore those situations, emotions, and/or persons that seemed to be linked to heavier drinking or abstinence. Ask what surprises, insights, or thoughts the student has had in reviewing his or her cards.
   a. *What was it like? What did you learn?*
   b. *In general, what times of the week do you drink the most?*
   c. *What people had a particularly positive/negative influence on your drinking?*
   d. *What things would you like to do differently? What's your plan?*

4. Give the student a copy of the feedback report and tell the student that he or she can keep it. Present each section of the feedback, moving slowly and giving background information when necessary. Elicit, summarize, and reflect the student's reactions to the feedback information (see section on Drinking Feedback, p. 86).

5. Ask a summative question: "I'm wondering what you make of all this. Where does all this leave you?" If the student indicates some interest in change, ask, "What would you like to do about this? What's your plan?" If appropriate, negotiate a plan of action with the student and/or provide a menu of options (see section on Talking about Change, p. 80).

Close the session (see section on Closing a Session, p. 78). If appropriate, arrange a follow-up session. Indicate that you (or designated staff) are available to provide assistance and support.

Motivational Intervention Session 3

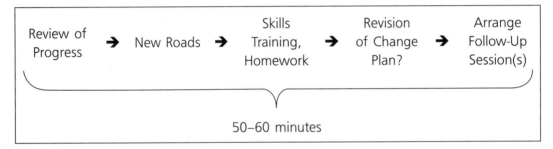

1. Thank the student for attending. Review material covered during the previous session. Ask the student how he or she has been doing since the last session, including (if appropriate) any slips the student has had with regard to drinking goals, what he or she learned from these situations, and what he or she would like to do differently in the future. Discuss times when the student was able to avoid high-risk drinking and affirm his or her efforts to remain safe in difficult situations.

2. Conduct the "New Roads" activity (see section on New Roads Functional Analysis, p. 88). Highlight the ways the student is using alcohol to achieve specific results. Discuss the specific effects the student is seeking or the contexts in which he or she typically drinks the most (see CEOA, Appendix E). Brainstorm (hypothetical or concrete) ways he or she might achieve the same results without alcohol.

3. Using the "Strategies for Low-Risk Drinking" sheet (Appendix H), discuss specific ways the student might minimize his or her drinking-related risk. If given permis-

sion, provide suggestions about drink refusal, social skills, relaxation training, and/ or drink monitoring (see Dimeff et al., 1999, or Monti, Kadden, Rohsenow, Cooney, & Abrams, 2002).

4. If the student will be seen for a subsequent session, ask him or her to complete the "Goal Setting" worksheet (Appendix N). Explain that you are particularly interested in what goals and strategies the student thinks will work for him or her. Encourage him or her to try out one strategy before the next session.

Summarize and close the session (see section on Closing a Session, p. 78). If appropriate, arrange a follow-up session. Indicate that you (or designated staff) are available to provide assistance and support.

Motivational Intervention Session 4

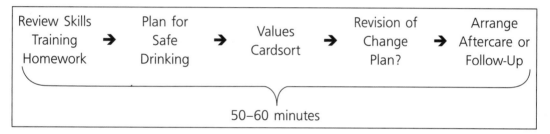

1. Thank the student for attending. Review material covered during the previous session. Ask the student how he or she has been doing since the last session, including (if appropriate) any "slips" the student has had in drinking goals, what he or she learned from these situations, and what he or she would like to do differently in the future. Discuss times when the student was able to avoid high-risk drinking and affirm his or her efforts to remain safe in difficult situations.

2. Review the student's homework sheets. Ask the student to elaborate on strategies he or she identified as ways to reduce drinking-related risk (p. 80). If appropriate, ask the student to elaborate on the drinking goals he or she identified. Reflect and summarize the student's plans.

3. Introduce the Values Cardsort activity (Values Cardsort, p. 91). Hand the student the deck of values cards (Appendix H) and ask him or her to select and prioritize his or her 10 most important values. Once the student has sorted the list, ask him or her to elaborate on specific items. Finally, ask the student to sort the cards into three piles that reflect the relation of the value to his or her current drinking. Reflect and summarize.

Summarize and close the session (see section on Closing a Session, p. 78). If appropriate, negotiate a new plan of action with the student and/or provide a menu of options. Indicate that you (or others) are available to provide assistance and support. Provide students with printed contact information and/or a map to the campus facilities that can assist them should they have further concerns.

KEY POINTS

- *Motivational interventions can have an impact on student drinking and reinforce safe practices.* Although they share similar core techniques, the motivational intervention builds on brief advice and behavioral consultation with much greater time for conversation and through exercises that prompt contemplation about drinking.
- No matter how "apparent" it seems, *do not assume that any student wants (or needs) to change*.
- *The first few minutes of an interaction are critical.* Use this time to build rapport and make the student feel more comfortable. Assume defensiveness or discomfort, thank the student for coming, acknowledge potential awkwardness, and provide a structure for the meeting. Ask open-ended questions and immediately reflect the student's response.
- Encourage students to examine the motivational "balance" of alcohol use. Ask about what, in their opinion, have been some of the good things and not-so-good things about alcohol.
- Present drinking feedback to highlight differences between the student's drinking and personal values or goals. Move slowly through the feedback, reflect the student's responses, and give additional information when necessary. Allow the feedback to speak for itself.
- Help students identify the *function* that drinking serves. Help identify new ways the student could get the desired effects of alcohol if he or she chose not to drink (or chose to drink moderately). Consider the New Roads exercise.
- Encourage students to identify a core set of values and weigh these in relation to current drinking. Consider the Values Cardsort exercise.
- Provide an opportunity for the student to track his or her drinking over a few weeks.
- End the session with a summary and invite the student to give his or her final thoughts. Thank the student for speaking with you. *Always end on good terms.*

7
Talking with College Drinkers in a Group

OVERVIEW OF THE CHAPTER

In the last two chapters, we outlined approaches for talking with college students *individually* about drinking. In this chapter, we talk about working with college students in a *group*. Groups are common in college alcohol prevention efforts. The reason is simple: Group dissemination is seen as efficient and cost-effective. American students are introduced to college life through group orientation sessions, educated in classrooms, and collectively graduated with words of wisdom from a commencement speaker. Likewise, in our experience, nearly every campus uses some group format to interact with students around drinking. Approaches range from large educational presentations[1] to smaller skills-based groups to groups that help drinkers process their experiences or garner social support for sobriety.[2] There are also clinical treatment groups that focus more narrowly on helping students who have already evidenced significant problems with alcohol.[3] In this chapter, we first review a number of limitations and difficulties in conducting groups and argue for an approach we feel is most likely to be effective. We then present several practical suggestions for leading groups. Finally, we make suggestions for integrating our suggestions into a one-to-three session small group. The purpose of the group is similar to the purpose of individual interactions—to motivate students to make healthier choices about their drinking and, for students who choose to continue to drink, to impart skills that will allow them to do so more safely. This particular model may be most appropriate for students mandated to attend as a condition of the student orientation process (e.g., residence

---

[1]Material for large-scale educational lectures is available at www.collegedrinkingprevention.com or at www.baccus-gamma.org.

[2]For information on conducting "process" groups, see Yalom (1995).

[3]For information on conducting clinical treatment groups, we recommend Velasquez, Maurer, Crouch, and DiClemente (2001) or Ingersoll, Wagner, and Gharib (2000).

life orientations), those who need to maintain official status within the university (e.g., fraternities, sororities, athletic teams), or those referred for a violation of campus alcohol policy (e.g., adjudicated referrals). This model can also be useful for students who self-refer with concerns about their drinking, though in our experience these individuals are relatively rare.

Groups can be complicated because of the variety of individuals present within all but the most selective assortments of college students. We cannot assume that all students in the group want to be there, are drinking in a risky fashion, or *need* to reduce their drinking. In fact, in our experience, intervention groups frequently consist of a mix of drinkers and nondrinkers. Sometimes this happens because an intact group of students (e.g., a fraternity or athletic team) is required to attend an alcohol education group. In other instances, individual students may be mandated to attend a group because they were in a room where alcohol was being consumed or were caught violating the campus alcohol policy on a rare occasion when they were drinking. In truth, facilitators will have to work with the group as it presents, whether or not individual members need or want the intervention. The group we have in mind consists of 5 to 15 students, ideally under the supervision of two facilitators.

Our suggestions for style and content come from two conceptual approaches: motivational and psychoeducational interventions. The first approach, the *motivational group* (Ingersoll et al., 2000; Walters, Ogle, & Martin, 2002), uses the MI style of counseling adapted for groups. As with individual MI, the primary focus of a motivational group is on increasing discrepancy and talk for change, usually through a combination of motivational activities and group process. The second approach, the *psychoeducational group* (Baer et al., 1992; Monti et al., 2002), uses didactic information and interpersonal interaction to inform and encourage students. These groups typically rely on content introduced by a facilitator, followed by discussion, training, and practice of new skills. Fromme and Corbin (2004) have recently provided evidence that a brief group format, combining motivational and skills elements, can be effective for both voluntary and mandated students. As you read this chapter, you will see that many of the stylistic considerations and activities described are borrowed from the individual approach of the last chapter. However, we must caution that groups are not a straightforward application of these principles. As we discuss below, when aggregating students into groups, additional dynamics appear that place special demands on the facilitator.

RATIONALE AND CHALLENGES OF GROUP PROGRAMS

Groups can be powerful vehicles for change. For most college students, drinking—whether responsible or not—is a social behavior. Thus, it makes sense that groups would be a potent setting for change, providing affirmation of safe drinking, modeling of appropriate behaviors, and relief from a student's sense of isolation that he or she is the only one making circumspect choices. In the best groups, members are free to share their concerns and fears, receive feedback, and practice new skills. Groups can also be more cost-effective than individual counseling.

Unfortunately, not all groups are equally beneficial. In treatment groups with *adult* drinkers, it is often the case that many participants want to attend the group, both because of their recognized need for treatment and desire for social support. However, when it comes to groups of college drinkers, let's face facts: Unless the participants are volunteers, getting course credit, or otherwise very motivated, most won't want to be there. Because of this, some participants may be reluctant to participate, unwilling to share honestly, or even attempt to derail the group through hostile or dismissive comments. In cases like this, groups can be much more difficult than individual interviews, and, in our opinion, less effective.

Two factors make it more difficult to conduct intervention groups (Diwan & Littrell, 1996; Walters et al., 2002). The first set of difficulties has to do with the additional skills demands that groups place on the leader. For instance, when moving from individual to group sessions, the number of interpersonal transactions is greatly multiplied. Not only must the leader attend to the statements and affect of individual group members, but he or she must also be aware of how *others* in the group are reacting. Further, group leaders need to be able to manage strong and weak personalities at the same time, perhaps simultaneously trying to contain someone who likes to talk while trying to elicit comments from someone loath to speak up.

The second set of difficulties has to do with the ways that people act in social settings. In the presence of others, there is a greater potential to defend oneself against real or imagined criticism. Groups amplify affect: Individuals may state opinions more strongly or introduce issues purely for the sake of bravado. Argumentative or highly resistant individuals can affect others through negative comments or verbal intimidation. These group dynamics may be the reason motivational feedback, a key discrepancy-building component of individual MI, can have the opposite effect when presented in a group context. For instance, if feedback is presented in a group of primarily heavy drinkers, there is the danger that there may be multiple instances of extreme scores, which reduces the discrepancy of the feedback. This may actually reinforce the "deviant" status quo; heavy drinkers may think they are in the norm, making them less likely to change.

The difficulty in navigating these pitfalls has led many to drift toward information-dispensing formats. "Unidirectional" groups that use primarily lectures, videos, and didactic instruction do avoid many of the problems that arise from student-generated content. But, as we have noted, knowledge dissemination models are a far cry from behavior change, and, in general, educational programs have not been effective in changing drinking practices in college populations.

These additional dynamics may also be the reason why, in contrast to individual approaches (Monti et al., 1999), several group interventions for high-risk or coerced students have thus far yielded disappointing results (Look & Rapaport, 1991; Sadler & Scott, 1993; Walters, Gruenewald, Miller, & Bennett, 2001; see Fromme & Corbin, 2004 for an exception). Some interventions have altered their structure to adjust to the group setting, either through combining group and individual efforts (Larimer et al., 2001) or by utilizing special group interactions (Darkes & Goldman, 1993), but for the most part, the effective interventions described in the literature and recommended by NIAAA have been individually administered (Larimer & Cronce, 2002; Walters & Bennett, 2000). Because of limited empirical support, the group intervention described in this chapter draws more heavily on our impressions and clinical experience in conducting groups and less on the findings of formal research trials.

You may sense our hesitation with groups, but we do not want to leave this section without giving the counter side. Groups can be enormously powerful vehicles for change. College intervention groups, if conducted well, can support moderate, low-risk drinking and healthy habits. Groups tend to generate more practical ideas than individuals alone. Groups can also hold members accountable to the decisions they have made. And, last but not least, the economics of group treatment require us to continue to work to find more effective methods.

STRUCTURE AND SPIRIT OF THE GOOD GROUP

Just as there are rules for participant conduct, we would suggest that there are rules for *facilitator* conduct in the good group. As with individual treatment, we suggest that facilitators employ the core techniques of open-ended questions, affirmation, reflection, and summary. Because of the complexity of the group, there may be times when a facilitator may not feel he or she is strictly following the motivational approach. Some deviations may be necessary, but the most important thing is to maintain the basic style of the approach through expressing empathy, reflective listening, and conveying positive expectations. More specific tasks include (1) establishing an agenda for the group, (2) maintaining an empathic, nonargumentative group tone, (3) assertively reflecting and summarizing group talk, (4) enhancing individual and collective discrepancy, and (5) monitoring and engaging key group members.

Establish (and Stick to) an Agenda

Structure helps manage chaos. For this reason, facilitators should decide early on what material will be covered and how long each section will take. During the session, the facilitator is a timekeeper, making sure the group moves from one activity to another and that conversation is purposeful (e.g., centered on the activity the group is currently engaged in). He or she also serves as the group historian, reminding members of past material. Finally, the facilitator provides a summary and transition between one activity and the next.

At the same time, by saying the leader needs to be assertive, we certainly are not suggesting that the facilitator result to bullying or dominating the conversation. Some benevolence and flexibility is required. For example, in a group of women, it might be appropriate to spend more time talking about protecting oneself against sexual assault or alcohol-related violence. In groups of athletes or Greek-affiliated students, it might be helpful to focus on ways that individual behavior reflects on the organization. Because each group is unique, it may be necessary to deviate from the agenda that the facilitator had planned. When this happens, the facilitator must ask him- or herself whether the deviation is in the group's best interest and likely to be helpful to its members.

Establish and Maintain an Empathic Group Environment

As we mentioned in Chapter 4, the "nest" for effective individual counseling seems to be empathy. This is perhaps even truer in groups, where the need to save face is amplified. We suggest that facilitators set an empathic tone by explicitly defining ground rules and by demonstrating empathic, nonjudgmental listening. For instance, at the beginning of the group, facilitators can take the time to make eye contact, smile, and welcome each group member. During the group, the facilitator should make every effort to affirm honest responses and opinions. The point is to make students aware that this will be a friendly and safe time. Early on, the facilitator should highlight the importance of confidentiality. Members will be much more likely to speak honestly if they believe that what they say will stay within the confines of the group.

Facilitators may also introduce ground rules into the group. Here are a few we sometimes use:

- Respect the viewpoints of all members. No student will be judged for his or her beliefs or past behavior.
- Be willing to participate in activities and share honestly about yourself. The group is an opportunity to reflect personally on information to make sure that future decisions are informed.
- Be willing to give feedback to others when appropriate.
- Share time with all members.
- Maintain confidentiality. Do not share what is said with anyone outside the group.

Avoid Arguing with Group Members

As with individual interactions, we encourage facilitators not to argue with participants. Although some amount of disagreement is healthy, arguments can also stall forward movement. Given two group leaders, one way to minimize the amount of unfriendly debate is for one facilitator to present material while the other occasionally gives an alternate (but still legitimate) view. This double-sided presentation mirrors the process of ambivalence that participants may be experiencing internally. In other words, students are less likely to argue because they feel that material is being presented *fairly*. This doubled-sided presentation also increases the chance that students will appropriately engage in the discussion. For instance, each of these statements, which might be made during a group presentation on drinking, has a counter side and could lead to further discussion:

- *Most college students drink alcohol.* However, most college students drink moderately, and many choose not to drink at all. (Review statistics on "normal" drinking practices among students.)
- *Alcohol is a depressant.* However, at low levels of intoxication, most people experience alcohol as a stimulant. (Talk about the biphasic effect. Ask the group to comment.)
- *Before entering a drinking situation, it is important to set personal limits on how much you will drink.* However, it is sometimes difficult to stick to personal limits when in a tempting situation. (Ask the group what things have been helpful in maintaining personal drinking limits.)

Because of factors we have already mentioned, it can sometimes be difficult to avoid arguing with group members who make argumentative comments or present inaccurate information. In some groups we have conducted, individuals have made, frankly, outrageous statements that we believe they would never have made during an individual interaction. (Our favorites are variations on the "If you're not getting wasted, you're missing out on the college experience" statement.) While some students may honestly hold extreme views, in other instances it seems clear that students are making statements not because they believe them, but merely for the sake of bravado. Such statements put the facilitator in an awkward position: Do you remain silent and allow the comment to stand, or do you confront the individual and risk an argument? We recommend that, whenever possible, the facilitator avoid directly contradicting group members. Because of the tremendous need to save face in the presence of others, Dale Carnegie cautioned, "Praise in public; criticize in private." While some individuals may be able to absorb a public reprimand, for others a public correction can have disastrous consequences. When threatened, individuals may indeed initiate an argument for argument's sake or start a debate that stalls the process and makes the group appear negative and unsafe.

As with individual sessions, a facilitator need not *agree*, either explicitly or implicitly, with everything that is said. However, it is generally better not to confront members directly. In some instances, simply ignoring a comment for the time being will give another group member a chance to correct the misinformation. In other instances, the facilitator can reflect the comment with a twist, reflecting only one aspect of the statement or slightly altering the speaker's language so that the comment appears more in line with the group's agenda. Another indirect technique is to reflect the comment, acknowledge that some people do, indeed, hold that position, and then ask the group for an alternate view. If it is more comfortable, one facilitator can acknowledge and explore the view, while the other facilitator remains more neutral. Finally, a more direct response is to remind individuals gently of the group purpose. That is, while the comment might be appropriate in another situation, it is off-track in this context. Here are a few ways to disarm resistant comments:

- *Well, you raise a good point. What about* [what the student has said]?
- *You said . . . on the other hand.*
- [To the student] *You said . . . and there are a lot of students who think that.* [To the group] *What do others think?*
- *Okay, so that is definitely one side. The flip side is . . .* (or, *What's the flip side?*)
- *I hear what you're saying, but in this context I think we need to stick to . . .*

Assertively Reflect and Summarize

As with individual counseling, the facilitator uses reflections to highlight individual comments or common themes that emerge from the group. Comments may indicate ambivalence, discrepancy about individual or collective behavior, or interest in change. In addition, many groups contain students who choose not to drink or who drink only moderately. As with the individual approach, reflections and summaries can be selective to some extent. For instance, in the paradoxical "Good Things, Not-So-Good Things" exercise (p. 115), more time is allowed for participants to elaborate on the benefits of moderate, low-risk drinking at the end of the activity. Other activities such as "Group Feedback" (p. 116) and "Group Values Cardsort" (p. 118) are designed to elicit discrepancy and talk for change. While there is no hard-and-fast rule about which comments to reflect, there may be many opportunities to reflect talk about the disadvantages of heavy drinking or the advantages of moderate, low-risk drinking or abstinence.

Reflections and summaries can be especially difficult when there have been disagreements between participants. When this happens, facilitators should assertively reflect and summarize the *contrasting opinions* of group members. In fact, to "cap off" disagreements, it may be appropriate to state that group members seem to disagree on a particular issue and move on. However, whenever possible, the facilitator should try to draw out points that the group *does* agree on. For instance, although individuals may disagree on whether there is an alcohol "problem" on campus, they likely would agree that, for many students on campus, alcohol *can* be a problem. If students can at least agree on this second point, this group consensus becomes a springboard for an "invited" reflection or inquiry about the kinds of drinking-related problems students typically encounter, how to recognize and intervene in difficult situations, or how students in the group can minimize drinking risks.

As with individual interactions, in many cases, the smallest fulcrum is enough to move a large stone. As illustrated in Table 7.1, even "weak" change statements can be reflected with a twist and pursued through summary and a request for elaboration. For example, in each of the cases below, the statement made by a group member is sufficient for a reflection and "invited" discussion of risky versus safer drinking practices.

The fulcrum in these examples is the suggestion, however small, that heavy drinking can have some undesirable consequences, or that abstinence or moderate drinking is a viable option for college students. The lever is the facilitator's selective reflections, requests for elaboration, and summarization. Movement happens when individuals identify nega-

TABLE 7.1. Examples of Reflected Group Statements

Statement	Reflection	Further query	Summarization
"I already make safe choices about alcohol."	"Sounds like you have developed a plan to protect yourself."	"What's your plan?" "What's your policy about . . . ?" "How do you manage . . . ?"	"Some of you already are making healthy choices."
"Some people on this campus have a real problem with alcohol."	"Drinking can have some real downsides."	"What are some of the downsides to drinking?" "Give me an example. . . ." "How are you protecting yourself?" "What's your plan to . . . ?"	"One thing that came out consistently was that drinking can have some real downsides and that it is important to. . . ."
"My drinking has sometimes gotten me into trouble."	"You're seeing that drinking can have some downsides."	"What are some of the downsides?" "What kind of drinking tends to get you in trouble?" "Tell me about a time when. . . ."	"Some of you mentioned some real downsides of heavy drinking in your personal experience."

tive aspects of heavy drinking and elaborate on ways that they might minimize their drinking-related risks. Discussions like these might, for instance, precede a skills-based component, such as training in BAC calculation (see Chapter 3) or drink refusal skills (see Chapter 6).

Enhance Individual and Collective Discrepancy

People consider change when they become uncomfortable with the status quo, whether privately or (presumably) in a group. As we have already mentioned, when moving from individual to group interventions, new dynamics appear. Because of the fear of verbal retaliation and the need to save face in the presence of others, members of groups can be much more reluctant to share their concerns or desire to change.

Fortunately, it is usually not necessary for individuals to admit that they are having problems with their drinking or are in need of change. This is especially true of college groups. In fact, we are convinced that the vast majority of attitude changes occur beneath the surface, with few verbal indicators that a student is changing his or her point of view. In many cases, particularly in a group, talk about others' drinking or drinking in the abstract can produce internal discrepancy. Furthermore, most of even the most resistant group members will admit that there are some drawbacks to drinking and generate strategies to reduce drinking-related risk, especially if guided by a facilitator who expresses empathy, highlights discrepancy, and reinforces change statements.

In addition to the motivational spirit that guides the conversation, there are several activities for building discrepancy in a group setting. Table 7.2 lists the pros and cons of some of these discrepancy-building methods. First, to highlight individual discrepancies in a group format, we have sometimes used a values cardsort activity like the one described on page 118. Second, discussions of drinking alternatives or ways to minimize drinking-related risk are often well received in groups. Likewise, specific skills, such as BAC calculation (Chapter 3), can be taught to groups with little or no resistance.

TABLE 7.2. Methods for Increasing Group Discrepancy: Advantages and Disadvantages

Method for increasing discrepancy	Advantages	Disadvantages
Brainstorming pros and cons of alcohol use	May raise awareness of potential drawbacks to heavy drinking.	Members may be dishonest in their responses and/or generate many more pro-alcohol statements.
Exploring the relationship between drinking and personal or group values	May highlight a discrepancy between drinking and values.	Members may be dishonest in identifying values or in indicating how drinking relates to them.
Brainstorming strategies to reduce risk (e.g., New Roads)	May raise awareness of acceptability of alternative strategies to drinking.	No likely drawbacks.
Giving feedback on *individual* or *group* consumption	May raise awareness of consumption as compared to national or campus norms.	If members are all heavy drinkers, may reinforce a heavy-drinking status quo.
Giving feedback on *others'* consumption	May highlight the fact that other students drink less than the individual thinks.	For most drinkers, no likely drawbacks. For abstainers, may highlight the fact that most students drink more than they do.
Giving feedback on other group members' receptivity toward cutting down	May highlight the fact that other group members would be receptive toward those who want to drink in a low-risk way.	No likely drawbacks.
Gaining a group consensus on support for abstinence or low-risk drinking	Most likely to produce lasting change.	Difficult to achieve.

Finally, most forms of MI use normative feedback as one mechanism for building discrepancy. However, unlike individual MI, personalized feedback on drinking has not yet been shown to be effective when used in groups. Examples of group feedback gone awry and the likely reasons for this effect have been discussed elsewhere (Walters et al., 2002). In short, the problems seem to stem from the need to defend one's drinking to others and the heavy-drinking norm that is created when aggregating heavy-drinking participants into a group. For these reasons, we recommend caution when giving feedback on individual or collective drinking in a group setting. More promising methods have included feedback comparing the student's perception of *others'* drinking to actual norms (e.g., "You guessed that 90% of students drink alcohol in a typical week. The survey said 60% of students drink in an average week.") or comparing the student's perception of social attitudes toward cutting down to actual amounts (e.g., "You guessed that 10% of fraternity members would be comfortable with a member who decided not to drink. The survey said 90% of members would be comfortable with a member who decided not to drink."). Still other groups have incorporated drinking feedback distributed *prior to* (Schroeder, 2001) or *after* group attendance (Walters et al., 2000). These processes may better benefit individuals.

Engage Key Players

When individuals aggregate, one tendency is toward "social loafing," assuming that other members will speak for them. Creating a safe environment, covering interesting and useful material, asking good questions, and keeping the pace of the group moving are ways to engage individuals who would otherwise be reluctant to speak. However, there are at least three kinds of individuals who require special interactions: those who are determined to derail the group process, those who are very reluctant to speak, and those who should be speaking because what they say will motivate others.

In our experience, some students seem determined to derail a thoughtful discussion of responsible drinking. These students may actively discourage others from voicing opinions through overt behavior and comments, by stating their positions with confidence, or by monopolizing group time (Diwan & Littrell, 1996). In many groups we have conducted, these argumentative, highly resistant persons have not only confounded the motivational process, but also supported a "re-norming" effect where deviant, hostile talk becomes the rule. In discouraging such interactions, the ground rules of the group should be explicit in prohibiting hostile or dominating speech. Members can be gently reminded of this rule. In dealing with hostile members, facilitators can use standard motivational techniques to handle resistance: empathic reflection, asking for elaboration on statements that are consistent with the direction of the group, and validating personal responsibility. Strategic use of simple time-out (e.g., ignoring argumentative comments) or differential reinforcement (e.g., attending to positive or nonargumentative talk) may also be useful in modeling a positive motivational style. If a person dominates by monopolizing group conversation, one technique is to look for a natural stopping point, summarize what he or she has said, and ask the rest of the group to comment.

Some students derail a thoughtful group in a more socialized and perhaps more entertaining style. This individual, whom we sometimes refer to as a "bravado drinker," is most often male and likes to brag about heavy-drinking exploits, complete with detailed descriptions of severe intoxication, embarrassment, and silliness. What makes this person unique is not his or her experiences, but rather the ability to tell good stories. These wild tales tempt other members of the group, and even group leaders, to laugh out loud in response. While the stories are often humorous, the obvious problem is that such humor and braggadocio tend to undermine the motivational processes we seek—an honest appraisal of the risks of drinking. In response, group leaders need to minimize their own laughter and gently redirect the group to more balanced discussions. This can be challenging when the storyteller is the most verbal member of the group, but some direction from the group leader is critical. In addition to simply not attending to the stories, group leaders can ask for alternative opinions and/or encourage the group to examine the genuine risks of the situation. As a final strategy, leaders can acknowledge that the story does appear humorous in retrospect, but that such stories can sometimes reflect genuinely risky behavior.

In marked contrast, other students are reluctant to participate. They may be uncomfortable speaking in public or feel intimidated by other group members. Yalom (1995) tells the likely apocryphal story of a man who attended a weekly treatment group for a year without uttering a word. At the end of the 50th meeting, he shocked the group by announcing that his problems were resolved and that the group had helped him enormously. Although rare, examples like this one suggest that it is possible for some nonparticipatory members to benefit vicariously from the experiences of others. However, in general, the more active a member is, the more likely he or she is to benefit. Invite these members into the discussion by asking them to share their personal experience. Pay attention to nonverbal cues that suggest that the person may have an opinion about something and pave a way for him or her to enter the conversation.

One additional group member should be noted. Especially for groups that already know each other (e.g., fraternities, sororities, or athletic teams), there are often individuals who speak with authority by virtue of age, experience, or leadership status. This person might be a formal student leader, such as a president or senior member of an organization. Many leaders, of course, come into their role more informally, based on social skills, personality, or reputation. If not obvious, listening to what other members say can give you a clue as to whom they view as a leader. If other members tend to agree with this person, nod their heads, or ask for elaboration, it is likely that they view this person as a reliable source. If this natural leader supports the aims of the group, we suggest allowing this person to make statements you might otherwise make yourself. That is, allow this person to promote responsible drinking practices, while you reinforce these comments through reflection and summarization. In some cases, it might be possible to meet with this person ahead of time to discuss the goals and direction of the group. Make this person the expert in telling you about the material and approach that would be most helpful for this particular group.

Avoid Aggregating High-Risk (or Coerced) Participants into Groups

In our experience, counseling with one resistant individual is infinitely easier than with a group of such persons, who seem to have an endless supply of resistant talk. For this reason, we recommend not aggregating high-risk students into a group. Likewise, groups should not be composed entirely of precontemplators, because, as we mentioned before, trying to build discrepancy in such groups can be enormously difficult. Students may be intimidated by others, fail to share honestly, and leave the room convinced that "everybody drinks." It may be possible to screen students based on motivational readiness or some other characteristic and then form groups based on this information. However, at this point, we have very little research to suggest how these groups should be formed or what the optimal combinations are. We are also aware that in many contexts (e.g., groups for students violating alcohol policies) you may not have control over how groups are put together.

Use Two Facilitators

All things being equal, we recommend that two facilitators conduct groups. At the same time, we recognize that this doubles the cost of the group. Thus, leaders will need to weigh the costs against the potential benefits of having another person to monitor and facilitate the group process. Involving two facilitators, rather than one, allows for more observation and interaction with group members. While one is expressing empathy and rolling with resistance, the other can be looking for and reinforcing change statements. Two facilitators can keep the agenda on track, help each other avoid motivational traps, and remedy problems should they occur. Involving two facilitators also makes it easier to deliver psychoeducational material. When covering didactic information, one facilitator can present the material, while the other offers an alternative view to present the material in a more balanced way. (Of course, disagreements between facilitators should be friendly and add to the forward momentum of the group, rather than detract from it.) Some of the very best groups we have conducted have been with cofacilitators with whom we kept up a running joke or banter. While one presented material, the other asked questions, offered occasional suggestions or anecdotes, and kept up a lighthearted dialogue. In fact, in some one-shot groups, where we saw multiple groups for one session each, we were able to script jokes and anecdotes into the group dialogue. Students always believed the stories were spontaneous and had a good time because the group leaders were having a good time.

Facilitators should meet prior to the group to determine if their styles are compatible, to set an agenda, and to decide who will be responsible for what portions of the group. Fromme and Corbin (2004) recommend co-leader teams consisting of one professional staff and one peer advisor; professional leaders appeared better at maintaining program fidelity, while peer leaders provided credible role models. We also recommend that leaders spend time debriefing after the group, giving each other feedback, and deciding on improvements for the next group.

STRATEGIES FOR GROUPS

As with the individual interaction, in the group activities that follow, we propose a sequence that follows a motivational style and flow. Early activities encourage honest discussion and group cohesion, middle techniques inform and motivate, and later activities shift the momentum toward a discussion of responsible drinking strategies.

Opening Strategies

Begin the session by introducing yourself and thanking members for attending. If the group is mandated or otherwise consists of students who are not self-referred, emphasize that you have been asked to conduct the group but that you have no formal connection with the campus judicial system (if indeed this is the case). Explain the limits of confidentiality and encourage members to keep group material confidential. Also explain (if appropriate) that you must report to campus authorities that individuals participated in the group but will not reveal specific information. Whenever possible, we recommend that group leaders be as independent and have as few reporting requirements as possible, so as to increase the likelihood that students will talk honestly.

Explain that your role is to facilitate a discussion about alcohol and to provide information they can use to make an informed choice about how they drink. The information you share may also help them decide whether they would like to make a change in their alcohol use, but ultimately it will be up to them to decide what (if any) changes they will make. While your institution does not approve of underage drinking, you realize that students have choices when it comes to alcohol consumption and that some students do choose to drink. For those who choose to drink, the intent of the group is to provide knowledge and skills that will allow students to drink in a safe way. The safest alternative is, of course, abstinence, and for students who choose *not* to drink, the intent of the group is to support these efforts and to teach skills to others who might be at risk. Explain that each individual plays an important role in helping other members make choices. For this reason, members are asked to share their feelings honestly and to respect other members of the group. As the group facilitator, you will try to encourage honest talk and supportive interaction, but will not argue with members about beliefs or behavior.

Ask group members to introduce themselves. You may also ask members to share additional information, such as:

- *What brought you to the group?*
- *Why were you required to be here?*
- *What do you hope to get out of the group?*

Group Forced Choice

This activity is used near the beginning of a group to set the stage for self-disclosure in a nonjudgmental atmosphere. It gives students an opportunity to voice an opinion about substance use within appropriate boundaries and to hear other students voice opinions that they themselves did not endorse. Before the group begins, write these words on pieces of paper, one per sheet, and post them around the room: *alcohol, marijuana, crack cocaine, ecstasy, tobacco,* and *heroin.*

Immediately after group introductions, ask students to stand and explain to them that they will need to move around the room for this activity. Point out to group members the various substances that have been posted around the room and ask them to physically move to the one that best represents their response to the following question:

- *Which of the posted substances is the most addictive (or dangerous) to the user?*

If any members seem to have a hard time deciding which sign to choose, explain that there are no right or wrong answers, and you are merely interested in their opinion. "Addiction" is defined broadly as the student understands it. Ask at least one person under each sign to share why he or she chose that substance and immediately affirm and reflect his or her answer. When every substance has been discussed, ask students to move in response to a second question:

- *Which of the posted substances is the most dangerous to society?*

Again, ask students to share their opinions, reflect the answers, and provide additional information as necessary. (If time allows, we have sometimes used an additional question, "Which of the posted substances is the most problematic on the college campus?") It may be appropriate at this time to share some basic information with students about the relative numbers of people dependent on these substances, numbers injured or killed as a result of use, and/or the economic cost of the different substances.[4] However, the purpose of this activity is to encourage students to begin sharing honestly in the group and to establish group facilitators as empathic guides who *will not argue with students.* When the activity is over, ask students to take their seats.

Group Good Things, Not-So-Good Things

This activity may be implemented in three different ways. Variation 1 is a straightforward version of the Good-Things, Not-So-Good Things activity described in Chapter 6; students brainstorm some of the pros and cons of drinking for college students in general. In Varia-

---

[4]See Anthony and Arria (1999) for a review of alcohol-related epidemiology.

tion 2, students generate lists of the pros and cons of drinking for them personally. Both of these variations work well for groups that are more cohesive or have evidenced some motivation for change. Variation 3 is a paradoxical brainstorm, in which students are asked to argue *against* heavy drinking while the facilitator argues *for* heavy drinking. This activity is useful for resistant or hostile groups and works best with two facilitators—one to debate with the group, and the second to support and encourage the group's efforts. We recommend the paradoxical version only if the facilitators have a good rapport with the group and can maintain a sense of humor about the experience.

Simple Brainstorm

Begin by explaining that people use alcohol for different reasons. Before acting, people often weigh the pros and cons of a behavior. Give each participant a blank sheet of paper and ask him or her to generate two lists: "Good Things" and "Not-So-Good Things" about alcohol. The lists need not be about the student's personal alcohol use, but can be more generally related to the pros and cons that students commonly experience as a result of drinking. When students are done, ask them to share their answers with the group. Write the responses on a board, overhead, or large sheet of paper. When the two lists are completed, ask the group to suggest ways that they might maximize the positive and minimize the negative effects of alcohol. End this activity by highlighting moderate drinking as a realistic option for most college students and a way to maximize the positive effects of alcohol while minimizing the negative effects.

Personal Brainstorm

This activity is similar to the "Simple Brainstorm," except that students are asked to generate lists of "Good Things" and "Not-So-Good Things" related to *their personal alcohol use*. After students are done with their lists, ask them to write a 1–5 point value (1 = not at all important, 5 = very important) beside each item to indicate how important that item is to them when making choices about drinking. Ask the group to suggest ways that they might maximize the positive and minimize the negative effects of alcohol use. End this activity by highlighting moderate drinking as a realistic option for most college students and a way to maximize the positive effects of alcohol while minimizing the negative effects.

Paradoxical Brainstorm

Tell students that they will be debating with you about drinking. Ask the group to generate a list of the positive effects (i.e., "Good Things") of alcohol and write the list on a board, overhead, or large sheet of paper. After the list is completed, tell the group that, using the list that they have generated, you will argue that college students can maximize the positive effects of alcohol *by drinking as much as they possibly can*. To get the discussion started, you might gently egg the group on (e.g., "This might be difficult . . . ," "This can be difficult for some students . . ."). Begin with the first item on the list of positive effects and argue for heavy drinking as if you were a typical heavy-drinking student. At this point, the second facilitator should emerge as an advocate for the group—encouraging the group to generate counterarguments (e.g., the downsides to drinking)—and keep track of responses on a second list. When you have finished arguing each of the items in the "Good Things" column, step out of your paradoxical role and affirm the group for generating a number of good counterarguments. To finish the activity, review the list of "Not-So-Good Things" that the group generated, ask specific students to elaborate on the reasons they identified, and reflect their responses. In this way, students finish the activity by elaborating on reasons against heavy drinking and hearing other students express additional reasons they themselves did not suggest.

Group Alcohol Pop Quiz

This activity is used to provide information and dispel myths surrounding alcohol use. Distribute the "Alcohol Pop Quiz" in Appendix K and ask students to complete it. Students should answer the questions to the best of their ability by marking each item "true" or "false." When students are done, discuss each item and present additional information where applicable about alcohol pharmacology, tolerance, BAC, risk factors, and consumption levels. Appendix K also gives the answers and additional background information related to quiz items.[5] When discussing alcohol-related consequences, it can also be revealing to show the graphical association between peak BAC and drinking-related consequences. If you have this information for your campus or the particular group (e.g., peak BAC and AUDIT score), consider plotting the scores on a graph and displaying it at this time. Information can and should be presented throughout the session, with or without the pop quiz. Present information in a nonjudgmental way and invite students to share their opinions and personal experiences. (Students always laugh when we suggest that they give themselves a quiz grade and mail the quiz home for their parents to put on the refrigerator!)

Group Feedback

Although evidence is strong that feedback can be an effective component of individual counseling, the evidence is more limited when it comes to groups. We are aware that individual feedback is sometimes provided in groups and has been described in one recent

---

[5]Aside from the material given in Appendix K, there are many excellent resources for alcohol-related information, including www.collegedrinkingprevention.gov, www.factsontap.org, and www.jointogether.org. The BASICS manual (Dimeff et al., 1999) also provides a wealth of material on the biphasic effect, gender effects, alcohol dependency, and harm-reduction strategies.

controlled trial (Fromme & Corbin, 2004). Yet our own efforts to provide feedback in high-risk groups have been difficult. There was a constant attempt to "abduct" the norm, devaluing general adult norms, and even general college student norms, as irrelevant (Walters et al., 2002). For this reason, we recommend caution if distributing or discussing group feedback on *personal* consumption. If personal feedback is to be included in intervention groups, consider having students complete the CHUG assessment (Appendix G) at the end of the group and mailing the feedback to each student.

Preface feedback by telling students that there are many myths on the college campus about drinking. One myth is that all (or nearly all) students drink. In reality, however, nearly 30% of U.S. college men and 40% of U.S. college women don't drink at all in a typical month. Many more students drink moderately, and it is only the minority of students who drink in a hazardous way. *Per month,* college students drink about as much as the average American adult does. The difference is that college students are more likely to drink in heavy episodes. In contrast, older adults tend to spread their drinking out over the week and tend to consume less alcohol when they do drink. This pattern makes drinking riskier for college students. (It also negates the health benefits that are sometimes seen in adult drinkers.) In fact, college women who report drinking four or more drinks in an episode and men who report drinking five or more drinks in an episode are at significantly greater risk for social, physical, and academic problems.

Continue by sharing the norms for your campus with students:

- The percentage of students on your campus who don't drink at all in a typical week/month
- The percentage of students on your campus who have two or fewer drinks in a typical week
- The percentage of students on your campus who report no heavy episodes in the past two weeks (i.e., those who did not consume five or more drinks in one episode)

Reflect student responses just as during the individual feedback activity (Chapter 6). It may be appropriate to mention the size of the survey from which these items are drawn, the year in which the survey was conducted, or the anonymous and confidential nature of survey responses. However, we caution facilitators against arguing with students about statistics. Rather, a simple reflection can sometimes capture students' reactions (e.g., "It's hard to believe"). You may also offer to provide interested students with written information about the survey at the end of the group.

Tell students that, given this tendency to overestimate drinking norms, many students feel compelled to drink because they think that *everyone else is drinking*. This perception can lead some students to drink when they don't really want to. If campus norms are available for the following attitudinal questions, present them at this time. If not, ask students to raise their hands in response to the following items:

- *How many students would be comfortable with a friend's decision to cut down on his or her drinking?*
- *How many students would be comfortable with a friend's decision to quit drinking entirely?*
- *How many students think a person can have a good time at a party without drinking?*
- *How many students would be comfortable helping a friend who wanted to stay sober at a party?*

Ask students who have raised their hands to elaborate. Affirm and reflect students' responses. Finish the activity by noting that the majority of college students drink in a responsible way and that the majority of even heavy-drinking students are comfortable with others who want to drink responsibly. Although there are many drinking options available to students, those who want to drink responsibly should not feel compelled to join the minority by drinking in a heavy or hazardous way.

Group Values Cardsort

As with the individual version of this activity (Chapter 6), this activity is useful in more cohesive or extended-length groups. Begin by introducing the topic of values. Give each student a deck of values cards (Appendix H) and explain that the deck consists of 70 potentially important life values. Flip through the deck and mention several. Ask students to select the 10 values that are most important to them and prioritize this top 10 from most to least important. When students finish sorting, ask if a student or two would be willing to share his or her list with the group. Reflect their responses and ask for elaboration on specific items. As in the individual variation of this activity, ask members to sort their cards into three piles based on how each value relates to their current drinking (i.e., my drinking helps me to get, has no relation to, or hinders me from getting this value). Ask students to comment on how they sorted their lists. To raise discrepancy, ask what differences students noticed between drinking and their stated values. Ask if a group member would be willing to share a time when heavy drinking interfered with one of his or her values (or how moderate drinking or abstinence fits). Reflect and affirm students' answers, particularly those that indicate discrepancy or intent to drink moderately.

With groups that have some initial motivation, this activity can raise awareness of the discrepancy between heavy drinking and deeply held values. On the other hand, we have also found that with some very resistant groups, this activity may actually solidify commitment to the problem behavior. As with the individual version, facilitators can ask students to choose a new list of values based on what they think their values will be 5 years from now. It is also possible to end this activity at any point with a summative comment, like "As students move through their college career, most find that their values tend to change. Things that seem important become less important, and things that they hadn't considered before become priorities. As you move through this process, I hope that you will consider how drinking fits into your personal list of values."

Group Problem Solving

Difficult situations often require us to act quickly based on limited information. Discussing the basic problem-solving process and brainstorming potential solutions can help students to make better real-life choices. For this activity, students are given different drinking-related scenarios common to the college experience: reducing risks, protecting friends, knowing where to go for help. This activity works best near the end of a group, in combination with instruction on harm-reduction strategies. It can be conducted in one large group or in several smaller groups that discuss their scenario and report back to the larger group. In each case, give students a scenario (Appendix L) and ask them to discuss how they might handle this situation. Tell students that in some cases, there may be more than one appropriate response because the scenario doesn't provide enough information to make a single definitive choice. If they are unsure what they would do, ask what additional information they would need to make an informed response and how they would gather this information.

- *What will you do?*
- *What additional information do you need before acting?*
- *How will you gather this information? Who will help you?*
- *Where could you go for additional help, information, or assistance?*

The scenarios represent situations common to the college experience. They are also times when students are less likely to make an appropriate decision—when they are in a group setting or don't have all the information to make a fully informed choice. Social psychology research shows that the likelihood of an individual acting in an emergency is reduced when many people witness the event. People fail to act in an emergency because they assume that someone, and particularly someone more competent than they, will act. Thus, the situation is doubly difficult because students must quickly gather information and act assertively when other students do not step forward.

- *You are at a bar with a group of friends. It is near the end of a night when you have all been drinking. You see a female friend about to leave with a man you don't know. What do you do?*
- *You are at a party and see a friend passed out on the couch. This is the first time you've seen him tonight, so you're unsure how much he's had to drink. What do you do?*
- *One of your roommates has been acting strange lately (stranger than normal), and you think it may have something to do with alcohol. He has been partying a lot and drinking more than usual at parties. While he used to drink only on the weekends, you've noticed that he seems to be getting drunk most nights. You've also noticed that he has been skipping the morning class that both of you are enrolled in. What do you do?*

- *You stop by a party to pick something up from a friend. You are there for about 5 minutes when you see an acquaintance with keys, obviously intoxicated, heading to his car. There are two others with him who also look like they've been drinking. What do you do? What if you were the host of the party? How (if at all) would this change your response?*

- *Your younger brother, Paul, is a junior in high school. You know that he drinks on the weekends and occasionally smokes pot, but as far as you know Paul has never had a problem with either of these substances. One night, your parents tell you that Paul has been getting into trouble at school, skipping classes, sneaking out at night, and has come home drunk several times. They also found a stash of pot in Paul's room, but they haven't confronted him about this yet. They ask your advice about how to approach Paul. What do you tell them?*

Ask students what plans they have developed to protect themselves and others when they drink. Pay close attention to comments from "veteran" students. Often such a person will emerge during this activity and be able to share valuable information with fellow students. It may also be appropriate to provide more information on alcohol poisoning, legal issues, guidelines for safe partying, and how to recognize an alcohol problem in fellow students. Describe services that are available to students who have questions about their own or someone else's substance abuse. Provide contact information and a map to campus services. Finally, if appropriate, encourage students to complete the handouts "Strategies for Low-Risk Drinking" (Appendix M) or "Goal Setting" (Appendix N) before the next group session.

SAMPLE GROUP INTERVENTION (120–180 MINUTES, OVER ONE TO THREE SESSIONS)

This section provides an example of how exercises might be integrated into a one- to three-session motivational group. The group consists of 5 to 15 students, ideally under the supervision of two facilitators. Additional activities, such as the Values Cardsort (p. 118), and/or personalized feedback (p. 116), might be included to increase the overall length.

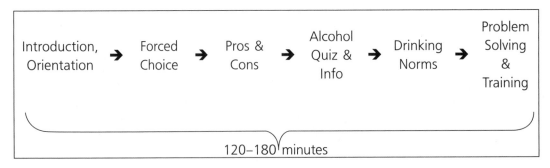

1. Begin by introducing yourself (and your co-facilitator, if applicable) and thanking members for attending. Give an overview of the group purpose, agenda, confidentiality, and any other procedural matters (see p. 113). Ask group members to introduce themselves.

2. Transition to the forced choice activity (p. 114). Ask group members to stand in front of the sign that best represents their response to the following statements. Reflect and summarize student opinions and provide additional information as necessary.
   a. *Which of the posted substances is the most addictive or dangerous to the user?*
   b. *Which of the posted substances is the most dangerous to society?*

3. Ask group members to take their seats and begin the "Group Good-Things, Not-So-Good Things" activity (p. 114). Ask what pros and cons of alcohol they personally have experienced. For a coerced or high-risk group, consider using the paradoxical version described on page 115.

4. Distribute the "Alcohol Pop Quiz" (p. 116) and ask students to complete it. Review the answers and offer additional information about alcohol pharmacology, tolerance, BACs, risk factors, and consumption levels. Invite students to share their opinions and personal experiences.

5. Present information about campus drinking norms (p. 117). Preface by explaining the tendency for college students (and even faculty and staff) to overestimate the number of students who drink heavily. Present campus statistics (if available) for the percentage of students who *don't drink*, who *drink only moderately*, and who *don't engage in heavy episodic drinking*. Reflect and summarize student responses. Explain how this perception might compel some students to drink because they think that *everyone else is drinking*. Ask students to raise their hands and elaborate in response to the norms listed on page 118.

6. Introduce the Group Problem-Solving Activity (p. 119). Discuss each scenario with the group or distribute the scenarios to subgroups of three to four individuals. Ask students how they would handle the situation, what (if any) additional information they might need to make an informed choice, and how they would gather this information. Provide additional information and/or suggestions as appropriate.

7. Provide students with a list of resources, contact information, and/or a map to the campus facilities that can assist them. Indicate that you (or others) are available to provide ongoing assistance and support.

KEY POINTS

- Alcohol prevention programs conducted in groups are not simple extensions of individually focused programs and have less empirical support.

- *It takes special skills to conduct groups.* Groups may place additional demands on the facilitator, such as having to manage simultaneous interactions between strong and weak personalities. People also act differently in groups than they do individually. Because of this, certain motivational techniques can actually reinforce a heavy-drinking norm.

- Early on, *establish an agenda for the group.* Some parts of the agenda, such as group content, can vary depending on the interests and needs of the group. Other parts, such as being nonjudgmental and maintaining confidentiality, are nonnegotiable.

- *Maintain an empathic group tone.* Make every effort to affirm honest responses and avoid arguing with individual group members.

- Use reflections and summaries to *highlight individual comments or common themes* that have emerged from the group, especially those that encourage low-risk choices.

- Enhance individual and collective discrepancy. *Use group activities* to provide a framework for discussing the risks of heavy drinking or benefits of low-risk drinking or abstinence.

- Consider groups that provide a *mix of risk and interest.* Groups made up solely of individuals with little interest in discussing alcohol are more difficult to run.

- *Engage key group members.* Use motivational techniques to roll with or reframe comments from those who directly challenge the purpose of the group or who fill time with humorous drinking stories. Facilitate participation of quiet members and encourage natural leaders to voice opinions you might otherwise make yourself.

- Consider using two facilitators to present alternate views. A double-sided presentation style makes it more likely that members will engage in the conversation without feeling they have to argue an alternate viewpoint strongly.

8

Service Integration and Training

OVERVIEW OF THE CHAPTER

Up to this point, we have talked about college drinking and its causes (Chapters 1 and 2), covered different assessment options (Chapter 3), and described strategies for talking with college students about alcohol (Chapters 4–7). Our focus has been on the details of the individual conversation—what to say, when, and how. In this last chapter, we broaden the focus to systemic and organizational issues. First, we address how the interactions we have described might be coordinated and integrated within a campus community. Although the focus of this book is mainly on aspects of the individual conversation, we do have a few suggestions for service integration, based mostly on consultations with colleges and universities. Second, we make a few recommendations for training others and getting techniques adopted into practice.[1]

HOW STUDENTS RECEIVE SERVICES

Conversations about alcohol are not exclusive to certain professions or providers, nor do they occur just once. College students can and, we believe, should be encouraged to consider their drinking choices again and again during their college career. Consider the course of a typical college male. He is oriented to the university upon entry, lives in a residence hall, moves to a fraternity, attends football games and classes, and has friends, resident advisors, and fraternity brothers. Alcohol prevention can be integrated into any or all

---

[1]For an expanded discussion of service delivery and evaluation, see Saltz and DeJong (2002). Also available online at media.shs.net/collegedrinking/FINALHandbook.pdf.

of these contexts. He may be oriented to campus alcohol policies in a large group, prior to the start of the freshman year. Periodically, during the first couple of years, he may be targeted by alcohol-prevention programs, such as alcohol awareness days, mass marketing campaigns, or educational lectures. When he resides in campus housing, he may be oriented to campus policies about whether or not he may possess, consume, or serve alcohol in the residence hall. If, at some point, he violates these policies, a resident assistant may refer him to a special group for violators. When he joins a fraternity, there may be new policies that govern alcohol use in the house. All the while, there will undoubtedly be faculty, peers, or health center personnel who come into contact with this student. If drinking-related problems become evident, one or more of them may encourage him to participate in individual or group counseling. The conversations we outline in this book can occur throughout this process, in both formal and informal meetings.

All of these contacts are types of preventive interventions. *Universal prevention* targets an entire population. An alcohol education program for all incoming students is one example. Other examples include social marketing campaigns, alcohol awareness days, and educational lectures. *Selective prevention* focuses on individuals based on their membership in a high-risk group. Students who join fraternities, sororities, or athletic organizations often receive special programs tailored to these groups (Larimer et al., 2001). Finally, *indicated prevention* refers to programs for those who have a specific factor that places them at greater risk or who are already having difficulties with alcohol. For instance, a student might be referred to an intervention after violating campus alcohol policy (Barnett et al., 2004; Fromme & Corbin, 2004). Through the lens of a preventive model, the alcohol-related infraction was an indicator that this student might be at risk. Other indicated programs focus on young people in the emergency room (Monti et al., 1999) or are based on an alcohol screening (Marlatt et al., 1998). There are pros and cons to each of these approaches. Universal programs have the greatest reach but may be less effective in changing drinking practices (NIAAA, 2002). Selective or indicated programs can more effectively change individual drinking but can be costly in terms of time and resources.

Aside from efforts to address students directly, there are often parallel efforts focused on environmental or policy changes. As we have already mentioned, college drinking is influenced by many environmental factors, including media messages, community norms, campus policies, and economic factors. Organizational-level interventions include collaboration with other campus, community, and judicial agencies to enforce local laws, monitor high-risk environments, deemphasize the role of alcohol on campus, and promote factors that discourage heavy use.[2] The Higher Education Center for Alcohol and Other Drug Prevention has recommended environmental strategies like the following to reduce alcohol and other drug use:[3]

---

[2] For an expanded discussion of environmental policies to reduce alcohol use, see Toomey and Wagenaar (2002). Also available online at www.collegedrinkingprevention.gov/Reports/Journal/toomey.aspx.

[3] For more information, see www.edc.org/hec/pubs/model.html.

- Working with local shops, bars, and restaurants to ensure that alcohol is not served to minors or to intoxicated students.
- Scheduling classes on Fridays.
- Keeping libraries and recreational facilities open longer.
- Refusing alcohol industry support for athletic programs.
- Restricting alcohol ads in campus publications.
- Monitoring fraternities and sororities to ensure that alcohol is not served to underage students.
- Promoting alcohol-free social and recreational activities.
- Disciplining those who violate campus alcohol or drug policies.
- Contacting parents when students engage in serious or repeated violations of alcohol or other drug policies.

Although these are all effective elements, they are not meant to be used in isolation. A better approach combines environmental and individual prevention programs in a multifaceted effort.

INTEGRATING SERVICES

Ultimately, we cannot tell colleges how best to fit these many efforts into their larger systems of education and health. Each campus is unique, and campus administrators must struggle with difficult questions about what services should be provided, where they should be located, who should do what, and how they will be funded.[4] Creating a responsive campus requires knowledge and competencies at multiple levels. The process often begins with a discussion at administrative meetings to identify people and services who might be interested in helping implement a program to reduce alcohol-related risks and communicating with other campus entities to ensure that efforts are coordinated. Getting skills adopted in more widespread practice involves clarifying who will be responsible for what aspects of different programs, training in specific skills, developing tracking systems, and making support materials available (Curry & Kim, 1999). Below we offer a few suggestions on integrating multiple efforts.[5]

First, train broadly. We suggest educating leadership in Greek houses and residential, mental health, and administrative staff about effective ways of talking with students about alcohol. Although training a few experts to provide alcohol-prevention and treatment services can be helpful, most college drinkers will never see such a person. In contrast, offering broader training to members of the campus community increases the probability that

---

[4]The Higher Education Center for Alcohol and Other Drug Prevention (www.edc.org/hec) provides many examples of effective campus services.

[5]For more information and suggestions about implementing organizational change, see Addiction Technology Transfer Center (2004), also available online at www.nattc.org/resPubs/changeBook.html.

risk-reduction messages will be heard, or at least that students will be referred to appropriate services. Of course, many campuses hire experts who not only provide direct services, but also training for the larger community. This model works well in many colleges.

Second, develop and maintain a continuum of services around alcohol use. One size does not fit all. The more options that exist, the more likely students will be to encounter something that helps them to examine their choices. We have described three individual models: brief advice, behavioral consultation, and motivational interventions. Models like these should be implemented where they make the most sense—brief advice and consultation in medical and academic settings where conversations may be brief and informal, and motivational interventions in counseling settings where more time and structure are possible. Yet, as noted above, prevention programs happen on a variety of levels, and it is likely that this aggregate effort facilitates the effectiveness of each of the individual programs. For instance, the results of a brief screening might motivate students to seek out additional information and services at a counseling center. Likewise, a social norms marketing campaign might reinforce the impact of personalized feedback provided in a counseling setting.

Third, campus providers should know what kinds of services *other* workers provide. For some colleges, this will be easy, particularly when student health, counseling, and housing services are located in a central place and under one administration. Other colleges that deliver student services through multiple locations and administrations may have more difficulty coordinating services. We suggest frequent meetings of a core interdisciplinary team to ensure that staff in different settings are aware of the range of alcohol-related services that are available to students. A group like this not only encourages collaboration, but links the promoters of a program with those who will implement it. As staff turn over and as programs develop and change over time, it may be helpful to set up other committees or electronic groups to share information. Personal relationships also enhance referrals, and thus, staff need informal times when they can meet. Although sometimes expensive in terms of staff time, an annual community meeting will ensure that providers know at least a few people in different settings. Knowledge of and willingness to refer to other services is critical to the effectiveness of a broad-based model.

Fourth, campuses should routinely screen students for alcohol problems. We know this is expensive and not in keeping with the role that colleges typically assume. Colleges appropriately treat students as adults who must be responsible for their own choices—colleges do not want to assume a parental role. There may also be a perception of legal risk—given knowledge of destructive patterns, a provider may be obligated to act on that information. While we understand these concerns, alcohol does pose a particular threat to the health of college students. This is a group at risk, and routine screenings can help identify those who are having difficulties and connect them with appropriate services. Screening also raises the profile of alcohol prevention on campus and makes individual students more contemplative about drinking. Screening can be implemented in a variety of contexts: academic orientation, health classes, or as part of health or mental health intakes. In this process, it is important to ensure confidentiality so that students' responses will not place them at risk for legal sanctions. For example, a drinking survey of incoming freshmen might be delivered by a campus health service, where the data can be kept as protected health information.

DELIVERING SERVICES AND FOLLOWING UP

In deciding how to allocate resources to address the problem of college drinking, we have given little space to the most intuitive method—decisions based on severity. It seems logical that students with riskier drinking habits should receive more intensive services, and many agencies organize services this way. Why have we not suggested brief advice for those with little to no alcohol problems, behavioral consultation for those with mild to moderate difficulties, and motivational interventions for those most at risk? There are indeed a few instances where we might automatically recommend a more intensive intervention, such as in the case of pregnant female drinkers, those who have a medical condition (e.g., diabetes) that is exacerbated by alcohol use, or those who are having significant physical symptoms because of their alcohol use. However, matching students to treatment based on most aspects of severity can be difficult in the college environment. First, it is difficult to know how severe the individual's drinking is without first conducting a clinical interview. All of our intervention models begin with an assessment for precisely this reason. The conversation—perhaps the *only* conversation the student will have around alcohol—may be well underway by the time the provider has any information about how severe the problem is. In practice, most providers will have to intervene with the student "on the fly." Second, despite the student's need, the reality of available services may dictate what he or she receives. The vast majority of alcohol interactions will not be delivered by an alcohol counselor in a controlled setting. Thus, we have attempted to provide models based more on available time and less on characteristics of the student. Third, and perhaps more important, there is very little data to support the belief that heavier drinkers benefit more from intensive interventions. Brief programs like the ones we outline in this book have been effective with college drinkers at both low and high levels of consumption.

We recommend a model of care where *successful response to intervention, or lack thereof, informs future decisions*. In a world of limited resources, the best intervention is the one that helps the student at the least cost. This means that we first try to intervene with the least complicated and/or least costly intervention and proceed to the next level only if the student fails to respond to the first. This "stepped-care" model is not new. It has been used to organize services in many medical and psychosocial contexts (Sobell & Sobell, 1999, 2000). For instance, in a medical setting, a doctor may diagnose a patient and, based on the findings, prescribe the least intensive course of action. If the patient fails to respond to this first step (or the problem worsens), additional measures may be taken. Likewise, if an alcohol intervention meets its goal—that is, if a student becomes more contemplative about alcohol or reduces his or her drinking or risky behavior—then no further effort is needed. If, on the other hand, risks persist, then it is appropriate to suggest a more intensive program or refer the student to a specialized alcohol counselor. For example, for the student described at the beginning of this chapter, one could envision a series of referrals based on follow-up to preventive programs. A peer in his fraternity might suggest he talk with a medical provider based on concerns about drinking risks. A medical provider could follow up with him after brief advice, and, if he is continuing to drink heavily, suggest that he see someone in the student health center who might provide a motivational intervention. What makes this method efficient is that the process can stop at any time. The student receives only the services he needs and is not referred from the beginning to the most intensive program.

Because it uses outcome to determine what comes next, *a stepped-care model requires follow-up.* We understand that follow-up can be costly and time-consuming. However, under the stepped-care model, additional contact is necessary to determine whether the intervention was effective and whether additional steps might be helpful. One option for contacting students after visits to health and administrative offices is simply to ask them to meet with you a few weeks later. Another option is to follow up with a brief phone call. At that time, the student is asked about his or her recent drinking and, if appropriate, given a menu of suggestions or information about additional services. If appointments are missed, follow-up calls or a handwritten note will make students more likely to contact you. In less formal settings, such as in a residence hall or classroom, follow-up conversations are often easier.

TRAINING AND EVALUATION

In the sections above, we have made a few broad recommendations for implementing effective campus programs. A point we have yet to discuss is training for those who will actually do the interventions. *Effective conversations hinge on provider behavior*, and thus, training should be a priority. Of course, not all providers learn equally. Like students, staff may be at different levels of motivation and willingness to adopt new strategies. For some, behavior change comes easily. Those who are already convinced of the need may benefit from user-friendly information, nonthreatening feedback, and ongoing problem solving. For others who are more precontemplative, it can be appropriate to focus on raising awareness of the problem, provide evidence for the effectiveness of motivational interventions, and draw out the concerns and personal advantages of implementing new techniques. For providers at all stages, feedback on positive outcomes can facilitate continued efforts.

Training for those who provide shorter-length interventions, such as brief advice and behavioral consultation, usually involves at least 2–3 hours of instruction, including a rationale for the intervention and instruction on ways to broach the subject of drinking, empathic listening, and advice giving. Given more time, providers can also be trained to conduct the Importance–Confidence Rulers (see Chapter 5) or other exercises, described in Chapter 6. Training in these brief models, like for all our models, is not just informational. There should be time to watch and practice the skills. As with training for longer interventions, role play is enormously helpful. For workshops focused on brief interactions, we recommend Allison's (2001) *Health Behaviour Change: A Selection of Strategies* video training and the accompanying book by Rollnick and colleagues (1999).[6] For standardized feedback on how a provider is conducting the interaction, the Behavior Change Counseling Index (BECCI; Lane et al., 2005), is a coding system designed to score the delivery of brief motivational interactions.[7]

For those who deliver longer interventions, such as MI, we recommend a thorough training in all the skills described in Chapter 4.[8] Although it is difficult to determine just how much training each practitioner might need, a typical MI training lasts at least 2–3 full days. Workshops usually consist of several elements: (1) didactic material on the theory and spirit of MI, (2) videotaped and/or live demonstrations, (3) general skill-building practice (e.g., empathic and reflective listening, rolling with resistance, encouraging change talk), and (4) specific instructions for conducting the sessions. After the workshop, we strongly encourage supervision by a trained professional. As a training aid, we recommend Miller and Rollnick's (1998) *Motivational Interviewing: Professional Training* videotape series. The Illinois Higher Education Center for Alcohol, Other Drug and Violence Prevention also distributes an inexpensive DVD resource focused specifically on college students, *Maximizing Brief Interventions for College Drinkers*.[9] This DVD includes several short video clips that illustrate the different techniques in Chapters 5 and 6. For standardized feedback on how the provider is conducting the interaction, the Motivational Interviewing Treatment Integrity (MITI) coding system is designed to score the delivery of longer motivational interventions.[10]

For those who conduct motivational groups, we recommend instruction and supervised experience in leading groups in addition to basic training in MI. Motivational and cognitive-behavioral groups place relatively sophisticated demands on providers, and thus we typically add 2–4 hours to talk specifically about *group* interventions. When conducting group interventions, we usually use co-therapy teams, pairing a beginning leader with a more experienced one. Because there is no standardized way to rate group interactions, facilitators are encouraged to provide guidance and feedback to each other. Each group is debriefed by the team, noting points of success and difficulty.

For all these training models, we cannot overemphasize the importance of practice and feedback. Many people believe that merely attending a workshop will be enough to

---

[6]For more information on *Health Behaviour Change* and other training videos, see motivationalinterview.org/training/videos.html.

[7]Information on BECCI can be found at www.uwcm.ac.uk/csu.

[8]Information on training opportunities in MI and a list of MI trainers can be found at www.motivationalinterview.org.

[9]For ordering information, contact the Illinois Higher Education Center, Eastern Illinois University, 600 Lincoln Avenue, Charleston, IL 62901; (217) 581-2019.

[10]Information on MITI can be found at casaa.unm.edu/tandc.html.

change behavior. However, in our experience, this is rarely the case. Although some people seem to come by the skills naturally, there is often a great distance between *seeing* MI and *doing* MI. Again, we emphasize that MI is a more a style, or *way of being* with people, than a set of techniques. It involves a *way of thinking* about the interaction—that students are ambivalent, that resistance is a natural part of the change process, that arguments tend to move a student backward, and that the student should offer the reasons for change. Of course, there are several factors that may make training more effective, such as a competent trainer, small workshop size (e.g., 12–15 participants), and a longer training time (e.g., 2–3 days), but we think the critical difference is that successful providers *practice* and *receive feedback* on the skills.

A final point of caution about learning MI: Although in most instances, we train all who want to learn, studies suggest that not all people learn MI with equal success (Baer et al., 2004). These data confirm many anecdotal reports from trainers that all learners are not created equal; for some trainees, MI appears to be easy, while for others it seems to be very difficult. If *style* is important to the success of the intervention, it may be important to select practitioners based on some criteria. Unfortunately, we have less data to suggest what the specific qualities or skills are that make an effective counselor. Our best guess, based on training experiences, is that the most successful MI practitioners are those who are comfortable with reflective listening and have a natural tendency toward empathy. Success with training may also have something to do with openness to considering other approaches besides an advice-giving or punitive stance.

FINAL COMMENT

We end this chapter, and indeed this book, by affirming those who work with college students around risky drinking. Your work makes a difference. Not all students drink in a heavy or dangerous fashion, but alcohol does have a long and deep-rooted history on campus. Given this culture of drinking, prevention efforts often have results that are difficult to see on a campus-wide level. It can also be frustrating to offer services that are not requested by those who will receive them. In our experience, few students actively thank us for our efforts, despite our empathic, reflective listening and support. Often a shrug and a raised eyebrow is all the feedback one receives that some contemplation has begun. In fact, if it were not for considerable research data in support of these interventions, we might hesitate to recommend them just from clinical experience. This is another reason service integration and follow-up are helpful. They allow you to see the impact of your efforts and gain support for hard work.

We are confident that, carefully used, the strategies offered in this book can reduce harm associated with drinking. We have presented several options for talking with students in ways that encourage them to think about their drinking, and, in this last chapter, we have suggested how these options might fit as part of a broad and integrated community effort. Input from students is, obviously, a large part of this effort. If we are open to feedback, students can teach us about their beliefs, perspectives, and choices and be active contributors to safer higher-education communities. Reducing high-risk drinking begins with an openness to, indeed a curiosity about, what students can teach us. For this reason, we begin our conversations with a request: "Tell me about your drinking."

KEY POINTS

- Individual alcohol interventions should not be used in isolation. Because of the culture of drinking on many college campuses, conversations should occur frequently across a spectrum of universal, selective, and indicated efforts.
- Conversations about alcohol are especially helpful when students are being oriented to programs, making an important transition, or being seen for problems that might be related to alcohol.
- To integrate campus services best, train broadly, maintain a continuum of services, facilitate knowledge and referrals across services, and routinely screen students.
- Follow-up assessments, although expensive, are necessary to evaluate the impact of brief conversations with students and to provide suggestions and referrals if problems persist.
- Thorough training—including instruction, practice, and supervision—is a critical first step in teaching people to provide a quality intervention. Training will vary with the experience of the provider group and the complexity of the intervention they are being taught to deliver.
- Keep up the good work and resist discouragement. Students will seldom thank you for prevention messages presented reasonably. Follow-up systems will help you see the benefits of your efforts.

Appendices

MEASURES

A. Alcohol Use Disorders Identification Test (AUDIT)   135

B. Young Adult Alcohol Problems Screening Test (YAAPST)   138

C. College Alcohol Problems Scale—Revised (CAPS-r)   144

D. Readiness to Change Questionnaire (RTCQ)   147

E. Comprehensive Effects of Alcohol Scale (CEOA)   150

CLINICAL EXERCISES AND MATERIALS

F. Importance and Confidence Rulers   156

G. Check-Up to Go (CHUG)   158

H. Values Cards   171

I. Self-Monitoring Cards   179

J. BAC Cards   181

K. Alcohol Pop Quiz   190

L. Problem-Solving Scenarios   195

M. Strategies for Low-Risk Drinking   197

N. Goal Setting   199

APPENDIX A

Alcohol Use Disorders Identification Test (AUDIT)

BRIEF DESCRIPTION

The AUDIT is a 10-item questionnaire developed by the World Health Organization to identify persons whose alcohol consumption has become hazardous or harmful. The AUDIT contains three questions on the amount and frequency of drinking, three questions regarding alcohol dependence, and four questions on alcohol-related problem behaviors.

TYPICAL APPLICATION

The AUDIT can be used to as a screening measure to identify people who might be having difficulties with their drinking and/or might benefit from a brief intervention or referral. For college students, we suggest using a cutoff score of 6–8. See Chapter 3 (p. 35).

ADMINISTRATIVE ISSUES

Time to administer: 2 minutes
Time to score/interpret: 1 minute
Computerized scoring available?　☐ yes　☒ no
College student norms available?　☒ yes　☐ no

COPYRIGHT ISSUES

Permission to copy?　☒ yes　☐ no
Contact:　　　World Health Organization
　　　　　　　Division of Mental Health and Prevention of Substance Abuse
　　　　　　　CH-1211
　　　　　　　Geneva 27, Switzerland

REFERENCES

Aertgeerts, B., Buntinx, F., Bande-Knops, J., Vandermeulen, C., Roelants, M., Ansoms, S., & Fevery, J. (2000). Value of CAGE, CUGE, and AUDIT in screening for alcohol abuse and dependence among college freshmen. *Alcoholism: Clinical and Experimental Research, 24*(1), 53–57.

Babor, T. F., Biddle-Higgins, J. C., Saunders, J. B., & Monteiro, M. G. (2001). *AUDIT: The Alcohol Use Disorders Identification Test: Guidelines for use in primary health care.* Geneva, Switzerland: World Health Organization.

Bush, K., Kivlahan, D. R., McDonell, M. B., Fihn, S. D., & Bradley, K. A. (1998). The AUDIT Alcohol Consumption Questions (AUDIT-C). *Archives of Internal Medicine, 158*(16), 1789–1795.

(continued)

Kokotailo, P. K., Egan, J., Gangnon, R., Brown, D., Mundt, M., & Fleming, M. (2004). Validity of the alcohol use disorders identification test in college students. *Alcoholism: Clinical and Experimental Research, 28,* 914–920.

Saunders, J. B., Aasland, O. G., Babor, T. F., De La Fuente, J. R., & Grant, M. (1993). Development of the Alcohol Use Disorders Identification Test (AUDIT). WHO collaborative project on early detection of persons with harmful alcohol consumption. II. *Addiction, 88,* 791–804.

SCORING

Item 1	0 = Never
	1 = Monthly or less
	2 = Two to four times a month
	3 = Two to three times a week
	4 = Four or more times a week

Item 2
0 = One to two drinks
1 = Three to four drinks
2 = Five to six drinks
3 = Two to three times a week
4 = Four or more times a week

Items 3–8
0 = Never
1 = Less than monthly
2 = Monthly
3 = Weekly
4 = Daily or almost daily

Items 9–10
0 = No
1 = Yes, but not in the last year
2 = Yes, during the last year

Maximum possible score = 40

A score of 6 or more is an indicator of possible risky drinking among college students. Eight or more indicates a strong likelihood of hazardous or harmful alcohol consumption in adult populations.

Alcohol Use Disorders Identification Test (AUDIT)

Please circle the answer that is correct for you:

1. How often do you have a drink containing alcohol?

   | Never | Monthly or less | Two to four times a month | Two to three times a week | Four or more times a week |

2. How many drinks containing alcohol do you have on a typical day when you are drinking?

   1 or 2   3 or 4   5 or 6   7 to 9   10 or more

3. How often do you have six drinks or more on one occasion?

   Never   Less than monthly   Monthly   Weekly   Daily or almost daily

4. How often during the last year have you found that you were not able to stop drinking once you had started?

   Never   Less than monthly   Monthly   Weekly   Daily or almost daily

5. How often during the last year have you failed to do what was normally expected from you because of drinking?

   Never   Less than monthly   Monthly   Weekly   Daily or almost daily

6. How often during the last year have you needed a first drink in the morning to get yourself going after a heavy drinking session?

   Never   Less than monthly   Monthly   Weekly   Daily or almost daily

7. How often during the last year have you had a feeling of guilt or remorse after drinking?

   Never   Less than monthly   Monthly   Weekly   Daily or almost daily

8. How often during the last year have you been unable to remember what happened the night before because you had been drinking?

   Never   Less than monthly   Monthly   Weekly   Daily or almost daily

9. Have you or someone else been injured as a result of your drinking?

   No   Yes, but not in the last year   Yes, during the last year

10. Has a relative or friend or a doctor or other health worker been concerned about your drinking or suggested you cut down?

    No   Yes, but not in the last year   Yes, during the last year

---

APPENDIX B

Young Adult Alcohol Problems Screening Test (YAAPST)—Brief Version

BRIEF DESCRIPTION

The YAAPST (Brief Version) is a 20-item test that measures personal and social problems related to drinking, either during a lifetime or in the past year.

TYPICAL APPLICATION

The YAAPST is used to identify specific negative consequences and difficulties that a student has had related to drinking. It may also be useful to point out benefits that the student might see from a reduction. See Chapters 3 (p. 32) and 6 (p. 86).

ADMINISTRATIVE ISSUES

Time to administer: 3–5 minutes
Time to score/interpret: 3–5 minutes
Computerized scoring available? ☒ yes ☐ no
College student norms available? ☒ yes ☐ no

COPYRIGHT ISSUES

Permission to copy? ☒ yes ☐ no
Contact: Kenneth J. Sher
                  Department of Psychological Sciences
                  University of Missouri–Columbia
                  200 South 7th Street
                  Columbia, MO 65211

REFERENCES

Hurlbut, S. C., & Sher, K. J. (1992). Assessing alcohol problems in college students. *Journal of American College Health, 41*(2), 49–58.

Kahler, C. W., Strong, D. R., Read, J. P., Palfai, T. P., & Wood, M. D. (2004). Mapping the continuum of alcohol problems in college students: A Rasch model analysis. *Psychology of Addictive Behaviors, 18*(4), 322–333.

McEvoy, P. M., Stritzke, W. G., French, D. J., Lang, A. R., & Ketterman, R. (2004). Comparison of three models of alcohol craving in young adults: A cross-validation. *Addiction, 99*(4), 482–497.

(continued)

SCORING

The YAAPST can be scored in three ways, depending on the time frame in which you are most interested.

To obtain "lifetime" prevalence: Score the question as 0 if the student indicates "Never" and 1 if the student indicates any other option. Add the scores to get a lifetime score.

To obtain "past year" prevalence: Score the question as 0 if the student indicates either "Never" or "Yes, but not in the last year." Score the question as 1 if the student indicates any other option. Add the scores to get a past year score.

To get a "weighted" past year score: Score each item as indicated below. This weights the items by frequency of occurrence. Add the scores to get a weighted score.

Items 1–6
0 = No, never
1 = Yes, but *not* in the past year
2 = Yes, 1 time in the past year
3 = Yes, 2 times in the past year
4 = Yes, 3 times in the past year
5 = Yes, 4–6 times in the past year
6 = Yes, 7–11 times in the past year
7 = Yes, 12–20 times in the past year
8 = Yes, 21–39 times in the past year
9 = Yes, 40 or more times in the past year

Items 7–20
0 = No, never
1 = Yes, but *not* in the past year
2 = Yes, 1 time in the past year
3 = Yes, 2 times in the past year
4 = Yes, 3 times or more in the past year

Young Adult Alcohol Problems Screening Test (YAAPST)— Brief Version

Answer the following questions as they apply to your drinking:

1. Have you driven a car when you knew you had too much to drink to drive safely?

   ____ Never

   ____ Yes, but not in past year

   ____ Yes: ____ 1 time   ____ 4–6 times   ____ 21–39 times

                       ____ 2 times   ____ 7–11 times   ____ 40 or more

                       ____ 3 times   ____ 12–20 times

2. Have you had a headache (hangover) the morning after you had been drinking?

   ____ Never

   ____ Yes, but not in past year

   ____ Yes: ____ 1 time   ____ 4–6 times   ____ 21–39 times

                       ____ 2 times   ____ 7–11 times   ____ 40 or more

                       ____ 3 times   ____ 12–20 times

3. Have you felt very sick to your stomach or thrown up after drinking?

   ____ Never

   ____ Yes, but not in past year

   ____ Yes: ____ 1 time   ____ 4–6 times   ____ 21–39 times

                       ____ 2 times   ____ 7–11 times   ____ 40 or more

                       ____ 3 times   ____ 12–20 times

4. Have you gotten into physical fights when drinking?

   ____ Never

   ____ Yes, but not in past year

   ____ Yes: ____ 1 time   ____ 4–6 times   ____ 21–39 times

                       ____ 2 times   ____ 7–11 times   ____ 40 or more

                       ____ 3 times   ____ 12–20 times

(continued)

5. Have you gotten into trouble at work or school because of drinking?

   ____ Never

   ____ Yes, but not in past year

   ____ Yes: ____ 1 time ____ 4–6 times ____ 21–39 times

   ____ 2 times ____ 7–11 times ____ 40 or more

   ____ 3 times ____ 12–20 times

6. Have you been fired from a job or suspended or expelled from school because of your drinking?

   ____ Never

   ____ Yes, but not in past year

   ____ Yes: ____ 1 time ____ 4–6 times ____ 21–39 times

   ____ 2 times ____ 7–11 times ____ 40 or more

   ____ 3 times ____ 12–20 times

7. Has your drinking created problems between you and your boyfriend/girlfriend (or spouse), or another near relative?

   ____ Never

   ____ Yes, but not in past year

   ____ Yes: ____ 1 time ____ 2 times ____ 3 or more times

8. Have you lost friends (including boyfriends or girlfriends) because of your drinking?

   ____ Never

   ____ Yes, but not in past year

   ____ Yes: ____ 1 time ____ 2 times ____ 3 or more times

9. Have you neglected your obligations, your family, your work, or school work for 2 or more days in a row because of your drinking?

   ____ Never

   ____ Yes, but not in past year

   ____ Yes: ____ 1 time ____ 2 times ____ 3 or more times

10. Has drinking gotten you into sexual situations which you later regretted?

   ____ Never

   ____ Yes, but not in past year

   ____ Yes: ____ 1 time ____ 2 times ____ 3 or more times

(continued)

11. Have you been arrested for drunken driving, driving while intoxicated, or driving under the influence of alcohol?

    _____ Never

    _____ Yes, but not in past year

    _____ Yes: _____ 1 time   _____ 2 times   _____ 3 or more times

12. Have you had the "shakes" after stopping or cutting down on drinking (for example, your hands shake so that your coffee cup rattles in the saucer or you have trouble lighting a cigarette)?

    _____ Never

    _____ Yes, but not in past year

    _____ Yes: _____ 1 time   _____ 2 times   _____ 3 or more times

13. Have you felt like you needed a drink just after you'd gotten up (that is, before breakfast)?

    _____ Never

    _____ Yes, but not in past year

    _____ Yes: _____ 1 time   _____ 2 times   _____ 3 or more times

14. Have you found you needed larger amounts of alcohol to feel any effect, or that you could no longer get high or drunk on the amount that used to get you high or drunk?

    _____ Never

    _____ Yes, but not in past year

    _____ Yes: _____ 1 time   _____ 2 times   _____ 3 or more times

15. Have you felt that you needed alcohol or were dependent on alcohol?

    _____ Never

    _____ Yes, but not in past year

    _____ Yes: _____ 1 time   _____ 2 times   _____ 3 or more times

16. Have you felt guilty about your drinking?

    _____ Never

    _____ Yes, but not in past year

    _____ Yes: _____ 1 time   _____ 2 times   _____ 3 or more times

17. Has a doctor told you that your drinking was harming your health?

    _____ Never

    _____ Yes, but not in past year

    _____ Yes: _____ 1 time   _____ 2 times   _____ 3 or more times

(continued)

18. Have you gone to anyone for help to control your drinking?

    ____ Never

    ____ Yes, but not in past year

    ____ Yes: ____ 1 time   ____ 2 times   ____ 3 or more times

19. Have you attended a meeting of Alcoholics Anonymous because of concern about your drinking?

    ____ Never

    ____ Yes, but not in past year

    ____ Yes: ____ 1 time   ____ 2 times   ____ 3 or more times

20. Have you sought professional help for your drinking (for example, spoken to a physician, psychologist, psychiatrist, alcoholism counselor, clergyman about your drinking)?

    ____ Never

    ____ Yes, but not in past year

    ____ Yes: ____ 1 time   ____ 2 times   ____ 3 or more times

APPENDIX C

College Alcohol Problems Scale—Revised (CAPS-r)

BRIEF DESCRIPTION

The CAPS-r is an eight-item questionnaire that measures the frequency of personal and social problems related to drinking in the past year.

TYPICAL APPLICATION

The CAPS-r is used to estimate the number of drinking-related problems that students have experienced in the last year. See Chapters 3 (p. 32) and 6 (p. 86).

ADMINISTRATIVE ISSUES

Time to administer: 2–3 minutes
Time to score/interpret: 1 minute
Computerized scoring available?   ☐ yes   ☒ no
College student norms available?   ☒ yes   ☐ no

COPYRIGHT ISSUES

Permission to copy?   ☒ yes   ☐ no
Contact: Tom O'Hare
                  Boston College GSSW
                  202 McGuinn Hall
                  Chestnut Hill, MA 02167-3807

REFERENCES

Maddock, J. E., Laforge, R. G., Rossi, J. S., & O'Hare, T. (2001). The College Alcohol Problems Scale. *Addictive Behaviors, 26*(3), 385–398.

O'Hare, T. (1997). Measuring problem drinking in first time offenders: Development and validation of the College Alcohol Problem Scale (CAPS). *Journal of Substance Abuse Treatment, 14*(4), 383–387.

O'Hare, T. (1998). Replicating the college alcohol problem scale (CAPS) with college first offenders. *Journal of Alcohol and Drug Education, 43*, 75–82.

O'Hare, T., & Sherrer, M. V. (1998). Drinking problems, alcohol expectancies and drinking contexts in college first offenders. *Journal of Alcohol and Drug Education, 43*, 31–45.

(continued)

SCORING

The CAPS can be scored in three ways, depending on the time frame in which you are most interested.

To obtain "lifetime" prevalence: Score the question as 0 if the student indicates "Never" and 1 if the student indicates any other option. Add the scores to get a lifetime score.

To obtain "past year" prevalence: Score the question as 0 if the student indicates either "Never" or "Yes, but not in the last year." Score the question as 1 if the student indicates any other option. Add the scores to get a past year score.

To get a "weighted" past year score: Score each item as indicated below. This weights the items by frequency of occurrence. Add the scores to get a weighted score.

All items
$$0 = \text{Never}$$
$$1 = \text{Yes, but not in the past year}$$
$$2 = \text{1--2 times}$$
$$3 = \text{3--5 times}$$
$$4 = \text{6--9 times}$$
$$5 = \text{10 or more times}$$

Items 1–4 describe *personal* problems related to alcohol use. Questions 5–8 describe *social* problems related to alcohol use.

Note: In published studies, the CAPS-r has used response options of 1–6, creating a possible range of 8–48 total points. For ease of scoring and interpretation, we recommend using response options of 0–5 (range 0–40). To compare the student's score to published studies, you would add 8 points to the total score.

College Alcohol Problems Scale—Revised (CAPS-r)

Please rate *how often* you have had any of the following problems over the past year *as result of drinking alcoholic beverages.*

	Never	Yes, but not in the last year	1–2 times	3–5 times	6–9 times	10 or more times
1. Feeling sad, blue, or depressed	☐	☐	☐	☐	☐	☐
2. Nervousness, irritability	☐	☐	☐	☐	☐	☐
3. Caused you to feel bad about yourself	☐	☐	☐	☐	☐	☐
4. Problems with appetite or sleeping	☐	☐	☐	☐	☐	☐
5. Engaged in unplanned sexual activity	☐	☐	☐	☐	☐	☐
6. Drove under the influence	☐	☐	☐	☐	☐	☐
7. Did not use protection when engaging in sex	☐	☐	☐	☐	☐	☐
8. Illegal activities associated with drug use	☐	☐	☐	☐	☐	☐

APPENDIX D

Readiness to Change Questionnaire (RTCQ)

BRIEF DESCRIPTION

The RTCQ is a 12-item questionnaire, based on the stages of change model, that assigns drinkers to precontemplation, contemplation, and action stages.

TYPICAL APPLICATION

The RTCQ can be used to assess motivation among drinkers who are not seeking treatment. It can also be used to determine what kind of intervention might be most helpful to the person. See Chapter 3 (p. 37).

ADMINISTRATIVE ISSUES

Time to administer: 2–3 minutes
Time to score/interpret: 1 minute
Computerized scoring available?   ☐ yes   ☒ no
College student norms available?   ☐ yes   ☒ no

COPYRIGHT ISSUES

Permission to copy?   ☒ yes   ☐ no
Contact: Nick Heather
                  Centre for Alcohol and Drug Studies
                  Plummer Court
                  Carliol Place
                  Newcastle upon Tyne NE1 6UR
                  United Kingdom

REFERENCES

Carey, K. B., Purnine, D. M., Maisto, S. A., & Carey, M. P. (1999). Assessing readiness to change substance abuse: A critical review of instruments. *Clinical Psychology: Science and Practice, 6*(3), 245–266.

Heather, N., Rollnick, S., & Bell, A. (1993). Predictive validity of the Readiness to Change Questionnaire. *Addiction, 88,* 1667–1677.

Rollnick, S., Heather, N., Gold, R., & Hall, W. (1992). Development of a short "readiness to change" questionnaire for use in brief, opportunistic interventions among excessive drinkers. *British Journal of Addiction, 87*(5), 743–754.

(continued)

SCORING

The precontemplation items are numbers 1, 5, 10, and 12. The contemplation items are numbers 3, 4, 8, and 9. The action items are numbers 2, 6, 7, and 11. All items are to be scored on a 5-point scale ranging from:

–2	Strongly disagree
–1	Disagree
0	Unsure
+1	Agree
+2	Strongly agree

To calculate the score for each scale, simply add the item scores for the scale in question. The range of each scale is –8 through 0 to +8. A negative score reflects an overall disagreement with items measuring the stage of change, whereas a positive score represents overall agreement. The highest score represents the State of Change Designation.

Note: If two scale scores are equal, then the scale further along the continuum of change (precontemplation, contemplation, action) represents the subject's Stage of Change Designation. For example, if a subject scores 6 on the Precontemplation scale, 6 on the Contemplation scale, and –2 on the Action scale, then the subject is assigned to the Contemplation stage.

Note that positive scores on the Precontemplation scale signify a lack of readiness to change. To obtain a score for Precontemplation which represents the subject's degree of readiness to change, comparable to scores on the Contemplation and Action scales, simply reverse the sign of the Precontemplation score (see below).

If one of the four items on a scale is missing, the subject's score for that scale should be prorated (i.e., multiplied by 1.33). If two of more items are missing, the scale score cannot be calculated. In this case the Stage of Change Designation will be invalid.

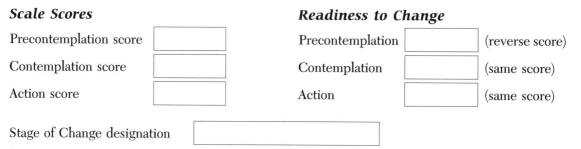

Scale Scores

Precontemplation score	____
Contemplation score	____
Action score	____

Readiness to Change

Precontemplation	____	(reverse score)
Contemplation	____	(same score)
Action	____	(same score)

Stage of Change designation _____

(Precontemplation, Contemplation, or Action)

Readiness to Change Questionnaire (RTCQ)

Please read the sentence below carefully. For each one please tick the answer that best describes how you feel. Your answers will be private and confidential.

	Strongly disagree	Disagree	Unsure	Agree	Stongly agree
1. My drinking is okay as it is.	☐	☐	☐	☐	☐
2. I am trying to drink less than I used to.	☐	☐	☐	☐	☐
3. I enjoy my drinking but sometimes I drink too much.	☐	☐	☐	☐	☐
4. I should cut down on my drinking.	☐	☐	☐	☐	☐
5. It's a waste of my time thinking about my drinking.	☐	☐	☐	☐	☐
6. I have just recently changed my drinking habits.	☐	☐	☐	☐	☐
7. Anyone can talk about wanting to do something about drinking, but I am actually doing something about it.	☐	☐	☐	☐	☐
8. I am at the stage where I should think about drinking less alcohol.	☐	☐	☐	☐	☐
9. My drinking is a problem.	☐	☐	☐	☐	☐
10. It's alright for me to keep drinking as I do now.	☐	☐	☐	☐	☐
11. I am actually changing my drinking habits right now.	☐	☐	☐	☐	☐
12. My life would still be the same, even if I drank less.	☐	☐	☐	☐	☐

From Rollnick, Heather, Gold, and Hall (1992), *British Journal of Addiction*. Reprinted with permission from Blackwell Publishing in *Talking with College Students about Alcohol* by Scott T. Walters and John S. Baer. Permission to photocopy this appendix is granted to purchasers of this book for personal use only (see copyright page for details).

Comprehensive Effects of Alcohol Scale (CEOA)

BRIEF DESCRIPTION

The CEOA is a 76-item questionnaire that measures individuals' expectations about what will happen if they drink, as well as estimates of how important that expected effect is to them. There are four positive scales (sociability, tension reduction, liquid courage, and sexuality) and three negative scales (cognitive-behavioral impairment, risk and aggression, and self-perception).

TYPICAL APPLICATION

The CEOA is used to identify reasons a student might be drinking. It can also be used as part of a brainstorming session on how else the student might get those benefits if he or she chose not to drink. See Chapters 3 (p. 38) and 6 (p. 88).

ADMINISTRATIVE ISSUES

Time to administer: 6–8 minutes
Time to score/interpret: 6–8 minutes
Computerized scoring available?   ☐ yes   ☒ no
College student norms available?   ☐ yes   ☒ no

COPYRIGHT ISSUES

Permission to copy?   ☒ yes   ☐ no
Contact: Kim Fromme
                  University of Texas at Austin
                  Department of Psychology
                  1 University Station A8000
                  Austin, TX 78712-0187

REFERENCES

D'Amico, E. J., & Fromme, K. (2000). Implementation of the risk skills training program: A brief intervention targeting adolescent participation in risk behaviors. *Cognitive and Behavioral Practice, 7*(1), 101–117.

Fromme, K., Stroot, E., & Kaplan, D. (1993). Comprehensive effects of alcohol: Development and psychometric assessment of a new expectancy questionnaire. *Psychological Assessment, 5*(1), 19–26.

(continued)

SCORING

The CEOA contains 38 unique items that ask about seven different factors related to alcohol—four measuring positive effects and three measuring negative effects. The chart below lists the seven factors, along with their corresponding number in the questionnaire.

Positive factors

Sociability
I would act sociable (38)
It would be easier to talk to people (31)
I would be friendly (14)
I would be talkative (34)
I would be outgoing (1)
I would be humorous (3)
It would be easier to express feelings (5)
I would feel energetic (24)

Tension reduction
I would feel calm (29)
I would feel peaceful (18)
My body would be relaxed (27)

Liquid courage
I would be courageous (22)
I would be brave and daring (19)
I would feel unafraid (20)
I would feel powerful (37)
I would feel creative (21)

Sexuality
I would be a better lover (32)
I would enjoy sex more (12)
I would feel sexy (7)
It would be easier to act out my fantasies (16)

Negative factors

Cognitive-behavioral impairment
I would be clumsy (15)
I would feel dizzy (13)
My head would feel fuzzy (11)
My responses would be slow (26)
I would have difficulty thinking (8)
My writing would be impaired (6)
I would feel shaky or jittery the next day (23)
My senses would be dulled (2)
I would neglect my obligations (9)

Risk and aggression
I would take risks (36)
I would act aggressively (25)
I would be loud, boisterous, or noisy (17)
I would act tough (35)
I would be dominant (10)

Self-perception
I would feel moody (30)
I would feel guilty (28)
I would feel self-critical (33)
My problems would seem worse (4)

To find *expectancy scores* for each factor, calculate the average score on questions in that factor from the *first section*. (Add all the scores for a particular factor and then divide by the number of items in that factor.) Use the following scale for the first section:

1   Disagree
2   Slightly disagree
3   Slightly agree
4   Agree

(continued)

To find *evaluation scores* for each factor, calculate the average score on questions in that factor from the *second section*. (Add all the scores for a particular factor and then divide by the number of items in that factor.) Use the following scale for the second section:

1 Bad
2 Slightly bad
3 Neutral
4 Slightly good
5 Good

It is also possible to find *overall* positive and negative expectancy scores by finding the average scores for all positive factors and all negative factors.

Comprehensive Effects of Alcohol Scale (CEOA)

COMPREHENSIVE EFFECTS OF ALCOHOL: EXPECTED EFFECTS

This questionnaire assesses what you would expect to happen if you were under the influence of alcohol. Mark a response from (1) for disagree to (4) for agree, depending on whether or not you would expect the effect to happen to you if you were *under the influence of alcohol*. These effects will vary, depending upon the amount of alcohol you typically consume.

This is not a personality assessment. We want to know what you would expect to happen if you were to drink alcohol, not how you are when you are sober. Example: If you are always emotional, you *would not* mark agree as your answer for the statement "I would be emotional" unless you expected to become MORE EMOTIONAL if you drank.

If I were under the influence of alcohol:	Disagree	Slightly disagree	Slightly agree	Agree
1. I would be outgoing	①	②	③	④
2. My senses would be dulled	①	②	③	④
3. I would be humorous	①	②	③	④
4. My problems would seem worse	①	②	③	④
5. It would be easier to express my feelings	①	②	③	④
6. My writing would be impaired	①	②	③	④
7. I would feel sexy	①	②	③	④
8. I would have difficulty thinking	①	②	③	④
9. I would neglect my obligations	①	②	③	④
10. I would be dominant	①	②	③	④
11. My head would feel fuzzy	①	②	③	④
12. I would enjoy sex more	①	②	③	④
13. I would feel dizzy	①	②	③	④
14. I would be friendly	①	②	③	④
15. I would be clumsy	①	②	③	④
16. It would be easier to act out my fantasies	①	②	③	④
17. I would be loud, boisterous, or noisy	①	②	③	④
18. I would feel peaceful	①	②	③	④
19. I would be brave and daring	①	②	③	④
20. I would feel unafraid	①	②	③	④
21. I would feel creative	①	②	③	④
22. I would be courageous	①	②	③	④

(continued)

If I were under the influence of alcohol:	Disagree	Slightly disagree	Slightly agree	Agree
23. I would feel shaky or jittery the next day	①	②	③	④
24. I would feel energetic	①	②	③	④
25. I would act aggressively	①	②	③	④
26. My responses would be slow	①	②	③	④
27. My body would be relaxed	①	②	③	④
28. I would feel guilty	①	②	③	④
29. I would feel calm	①	②	③	④
30. I would feel moody	①	②	③	④
31. It would be easier to talk to people	①	②	③	④
32. I would be a better lover	①	②	③	④
33. I would feel self-critical	①	②	③	④
34. I would be talkative	①	②	③	④
35. I would act tough	①	②	③	④
36. I would take risks	①	②	③	④
37. I would feel powerful	①	②	③	④
38. I would act sociable	①	②	③	④

COMPREHENSIVE EFFECTS OF ALCOHOL: EVALUATIONS

This questionnaire assesses whether you think each effect, which may result from drinking alcohol, is bad or good.

Mark a response number from 1, for bad, to 5, for good—depending on whether you think this particular effect is bad, neutral, or good, etc.

We want to know if you think a particular effect is bad or good, REGARDLESS of whether you expect it to happen to YOU personally when you drink alcohol.

This effect of alcohol is:	Bad	Slightly bad	Neutral	Slightly good	Good
1. Being outgoing	①	②	③	④	⑤
2. Dulled senses	①	②	③	④	⑤
3. Being humorous	①	②	③	④	⑤
4. Problems seeming worse	①	②	③	④	⑤
5. Expressing feelings more easily	①	②	③	④	⑤
6. Impaired writing	①	②	③	④	⑤
7. Feeling sexy	①	②	③	④	⑤
8. Having difficulty thinking	①	②	③	④	⑤
9. Neglecting obligations	①	②	③	④	⑤
10. Being dominant	①	②	③	④	⑤

(continued)

Comprehensive Effects of Alcohol Scale (CEOA) *(page 3 of 3)*

This effect of alcohol is:	Bad	Slightly bad	Neutral	Slightly good	Good
11. Head feeling fuzzy	①	②	③	④	⑤
12. Enjoying sex more	①	②	③	④	⑤
13. Feeling dizzy	①	②	③	④	⑤
14. Being friendly	①	②	③	④	⑤
15. Being clumsy	①	②	③	④	⑤
16. Easier to act out fantasies	①	②	③	④	⑤
17. Being loud, boisterous, or noisy	①	②	③	④	⑤
18. Feeling peaceful	①	②	③	④	⑤
19. Being brave and daring	①	②	③	④	⑤
20. Feeling unafraid	①	②	③	④	⑤
21. Feeling creative	①	②	③	④	⑤
22. Being courageous	①	②	③	④	⑤
23. Feeling shaky or jittery the next day	①	②	③	④	⑤
24. Feeling energetic	①	②	③	④	⑤
25. Acting aggressively	①	②	③	④	⑤
26. Having slow responses	①	②	③	④	⑤
27. Having a relaxed body	①	②	③	④	⑤
28. Feeling guilty	①	②	③	④	⑤
29. Feeling calm	①	②	③	④	⑤
30. Feeling moody	①	②	③	④	⑤
31. Being easier to talk to people	①	②	③	④	⑤
32. Being a better lover	①	②	③	④	⑤
33. Feeling self-critical	①	②	③	④	⑤
34. Being talkative	①	②	③	④	⑤
35. Acting tough	①	②	③	④	⑤
36. Taking risks	①	②	③	④	⑤
37. Feeling powerful	①	②	③	④	⑤
38. Acting sociable	①	②	③	④	⑤

APPENDIX F

Importance and Confidence Rulers

BRIEF DESCRIPTION

The Importance and Confidence Rulers are scaled questions that ask how important a change is and how confident the person is that he or she could change if he or she wanted to.

TYPICAL APPLICATION

The Importance and Confidence Rulers are used to assess levels of motivation, to inform treatment approach, and as a brief motivational technique for encouraging the student to talk about change. See Chapters 3 (p. 37) and 5 (p. 67).

ADMINISTRATIVE ISSUES

Time to administer: 1–10 minutes
Time to score/interpret: n/a
Computerized scoring available?　☐ yes　☒ no
College student norms available?　☐ yes　☒ no

COPYRIGHT ISSUES

Permission to copy?　☒ yes　☐ no

REFERENCES

Miller, W. R., & Rollnick, S. (2002). *Motivational interviewing: Preparing people for change* (2nd ed.). New York: Guilford Press.
Rollnick, S., Mason, P., & Butler, C. (1999). *Health behavior change: A guide for practitioners*. Edinburgh, UK: Churchill Livingstone.

Importance and Confidence Rulers

IMPORTANCE RULER

On a scale of 1–10, how important is it for you to make a change in your drinking?

| 1 | 2 | 3 | 4 | 5 | 6 | 7 | 8 | 9 | 10 |

←——————————————————————————————————→

Not at all important   Extremely important

CONFIDENCE RULER

On a scale of 1–10, how confident are you that you could make a change if you wanted to?

| 1 | 2 | 3 | 4 | 5 | 6 | 7 | 8 | 9 | 10 |

←——————————————————————————————————→

Not at all confident   Extremely confident

Adapted from Miller and Rollnick (2002). Copyright 2002 by The Guilford Press. Reprinted with permission in *Talking with College Students about Alcohol* by Scott T. Walters and John S. Baer. Permission to photocopy this appendix is granted to purchasers of this book for personal use only (see copyright page for details).

APPENDIX G

Check-Up to Go (CHUG)

BRIEF DESCRIPTION

The CHUG assesses and provides feedback to students on alcohol consumption, potential risk factors, and comparison to college norms.

TYPICAL APPLICATION

Feedback from the CHUG can be mailed to students or presented as part of an individual or group counseling session. See Chapters 6 (p. 86) and 7 (p. 117).

ADMINISTRATIVE ISSUES

Time to administer: 5–10 minutes
Time to score/interpret: 10–15 minutes
Computerized scoring available?   ☒ yes   ☐ no
College student norms available?   ☐ yes   ☒ no

COPYRIGHT ISSUES

Permission to copy?   ☒ yes   ☐ no
Contact: Scott Walters
                  University of Texas School of Public Health
                  Dallas Regional Campus
                  5323 Harry Hines Boulevard, V8.112
                  Dallas, TX 75390-9128

REFERENCES

Walters, S. T. (2000). In praise of feedback: An effective intervention for college students who are heavy drinkers. *Journal of American College Health, 48,* 235–238.

Walters, S. T., Bennett, M. E., & Miller. J. E. (2000). Reducing alcohol use in college students: A controlled trial of two brief interventions. *Journal of Drug Education, 30*(3), 361–372.

Walters, S. T., Gruenewald, D. A., Miller, J. H., & Bennett, M. E. (2001). Early findings from a disciplinary program to reduce problem drinking by college students. *Journal of Substance Abuse Treatment, 20*(1), 89–91.

Walters, S. T., & Woodall, W. G. (2003). Mailed feedback reduces consumption among moderate drinkers who are employed. *Prevention Science, 4*(4), 287–294.

See also www.e-chug.com.

✓ *Check-Up to Go*

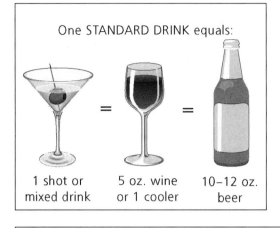

One STANDARD DRINK equals:

= =

1 shot or mixed drink
5 oz. wine or 1 cooler
10–12 oz. beer

In order to provide you with the most accurate feedback, please answer the following questions honestly. Remember that your answers are CONFIDENTIAL. Please put your name and mailing address below:

_____

_____

_____

_____

_____

What is your gender? _____ Weight? _____ Currently taking prescription medications? _____

1. For the PAST MONTH, please describe a TYPICAL DRINKING WEEK. For each day, fill in the number of STANDARD DRINKS of each type of alcohol you consumed on that day and the TYPICAL NUMBER OF HOURS you drank on that day.

	Mon.	Tues.	Wed.	Thurs.	Fri.	Sat.	Sun.
BEER?							
WINE?							
SPIRITS?							
HOURS?							

2. Think of the one occasion during the PAST MONTH when you drank the most. Fill in the number of standard drinks of each type you consumed.

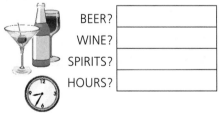

BEER?	
WINE?	
SPIRITS?	
HOURS?	

3. Think about the number of your BLOOD RELATIVES who are now, or have been in the past, problem drinkers or alcoholics.

NUMBER

Number of parents? _____

Number of brothers or sisters? _____

Number of grandparents? _____

Number of uncles or aunts? _____

Number of first cousins? _____

4. During the PAST MONTH, how many days did you drive a vehicle shortly after having three or more drinks? . . . . [ ]

5. During the PAST MONTH, how many days were you a passenger in a vehicle when the driver had three or more drinks? . . . . [ ]

6. How much would you estimate you spend on alcoholic beverages per week? . . . . . . [$]

7. For each of the following, estimate how common these behaviors are:

   What percent of U.S. college students (same sex) drink more than you? . . . . [ ]

   What percent of U.S. college students do not drink at all in a typical week? . . . . [ ]

   What percent of U.S. college students have two drinks or fewer in a typical week? . . . [ ]

   What percent of U.S. college students smoke marijuana at least once a year? . . . . [ ]

---

8. Please circle the answer that is correct for you:

   a. How often do you have a drink containing alcohol?

Never	Monthly or less	Two to four times a month	Two to three times a week	Four or more times a week

   b. How many drinks containing alcohol do you have on a typical day when you are drinking?

1 or 2	3 or 4	5 or 6	7 to 9	10 or more

   c. How often do you have six drinks or more on one occasion?

Never	Less than monthly	Monthly	Weekly	Daily or almost daily

   d. How often during the last year have you found that you were not able to stop drinking once you had started?

Never	Less than monthly	Monthly	Weekly	Daily or almost daily

   e. How often during the last year have you failed to do what was normally expected from you because of drinking?

Never	Less than monthly	Monthly	Weekly	Daily or almost daily

   f. How often during the last year have you needed a first drink in the morning to get yourself going after a heavy drinking session?

Never	Less than monthly	Monthly	Weekly	Daily or almost daily

   g. How often during the last year have you had a feeling of guilt or remorse after drinking?

Never	Less than monthly	Monthly	Weekly	Daily or almost daily

(continued)

h. How often during the last year have you been unable to remember what happened the night before because you had been drinking?

Never   Less than   Monthly   Weekly   Daily or
               monthly   almost daily

i. Have you or someone else been injured as a result of your drinking?

No   Yes, but not in the last year   Yes, during the last year

j. Has a relative or friend or a doctor or other health worker been concerned about your drinking or suggested you cut down?

No   Yes, but not in the last year   Yes, during the last year

AUDIT. World Health Organization. Used by permission.

9. During the PAST MONTH, how many cigarettes did you smoke on a typical day? . . . . .

10. If a smoker, for how many years have you smoked regularly? . . . .

11. After school expenses, how much money do you have to spend in an average month? . . . . $

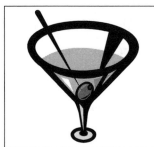

Your personal profile from the

Check-Up to Go

#1 Your Drinking Profile

Standard drinks per month _____

Standard drinks per week _____

Amount spent on alcohol per year $_____

Percent of spending money used to buy alcohol _____%

These are the average number of drinks that you reported having in a typical month and week. Also listed is the percent of income that you reported spending on alcohol and the total spent per year. Because alcoholic beverages vary in strength, we have converted your drinking pattern into standard units. In this system, "one drink" equals:

12 oz. beer = 5 oz. wine = 1 shot or mixed drink

Percent of American adults (same sex) who drink less than you: _____%

This number, based on the National Alcohol Survey, tells you what percent of U.S. men (if you are a man) or women (if you are a woman) drink less than you in a typical week.

How much is too much? Research indicates that college men who have four or fewer drinks when they drink, and women who have three or fewer drinks when they drink, have fewer health, academic, and social problems.

For some people, however, even 1–2 drinks per day is too many. Pregnant women, for example, are best advised to abstain from alcohol altogether because even small amounts have been found to increase risk to the unborn child. Some health problems (such as liver disease) make even moderate drinking unsafe. Other people find that they are unable to drink moderately, and having even one or two drinks leads to feeling intoxicated.

Your total number of drinks per week tells only part of the story. It is not healthy, for example, to have 12 drinks per week by saving them all up for Saturday. Neither is it safe to have even a couple of drinks and then drive.

#2 Level of Intoxication

Estimated highest blood alcohol concentration *during a typical week:* _____%

Estimated highest blood alcohol concentration *during your heaviest drinking episode:* _____%

A second way of looking at your drinking is in terms of your peak level of intoxication. Blood alcohol concentration (BAC) is an indicator of the extent to which alcohol is affecting your body and behavior. **BAC is like a thermometer—the higher it is, the greater the intoxication.** How high your BAC gets depends on your weight, the strength and number of drinks you have, and how quickly you drink.

These factors might result in **a *higher* BAC level** than you would otherwise expect:

- Drinking on an empty stomach
- Using alcohol in combination with other drugs
- Being on a diet or under your normal weight
- Certain emotional states or menstrual cycle phase
- Being fatigued, dehydrated, or recently ill

One factor that might result in **a *lower* BAC** than you would otherwise expect is eating food before and while drinking.

Factors that ***do not affect* BAC** include:

- Coffee and other stimulants
- Exercise, a cold shower, or a walk
- Fruit juices or special concoctions

Your body gets rid of alcohol at a relatively constant rate of about one standard drink per hour. There is nothing that you can do to speed up this process of elimination once alcohol is in your bloodstream.

Research note: Alcohol-related physical problems are strongly related to the number of heavy drinking occasions. Heavy drinking once or twice a week may cause more damage than smaller amounts over several days.

BAC Levels		
.02% Light and moderate drinkers begin to feel relaxed. Driving, even at this level, can be risky. In most states it is illegal for those under 21 to drive at this BAC level.	**.10%** Reaction time and muscle control are impaired. This level is considered legally drunk in all 50 states. A person driving at this level is 10 times more likely to cause a fatal accident. Normal social drinkers rarely reach this level.	**.30%** Many people lose consciousness, either falling asleep or passing out. Individuals who have a high tolerance to alcohol may remain conscious at much higher BAC levels. Such a high tolerance is a serious risk factor for health problems.
.04% Most drinkers begin to feel relaxed. (Rapid drinking can create the illusion that it takes more alcohol to feel relaxed because the first drinks are taking effect while later drinks are being consumed). Most normal drinkers taper off their drinking between .04 and .06. (For women who are pregnant, there is no safe level of alcohol consumption. Even moderate drinking can place an unborn child at risk.)	**.12%** Vomiting occurs in a normal person unless the drinker has reached this level gradually or has a substantial tolerance to alcohol. Vomiting is a normal protective reaction of the body.	**.40%** Most people lose consciousness, a protective reaction that prevents the person from continuing to drink. Risk of death from alcohol poisoning begins to increase.
.06% Judgment is somewhat impaired. People are less likely to make sound judgments about their capabilities (like ability to drive safely). This BAC level is considered legally intoxicated in some states.	**.15%** Balance and movement are substantially impaired. The person has difficulty walking or talking in a normal fashion. Heavy drinkers with a substantial tolerance to alcohol may learn to look sober at this level, though in fact they are intoxicated. This level means that the equivalent of approximately one half pint of whiskey is circulating in the bloodstream. A person driving at this level is 25 times more likely to cause a fatal accident.	**.45%** This is a fatal dose for about half of normal individuals. Alcohol at this level can paralyze the part of the brain that controls breathing and heart rate. Vital functions cease and the person dies of respiratory or cardiovascular failure. This can happen when someone drinks a large amount of alcohol, passes out, and the alcohol in the stomach continues to be absorbed into the bloodstream, causing a fatal dose. This is a special danger in drinking contests, a frequent cause of lethal overdose among young drinkers.
.08% Judgment is further impaired. People are more likely to do things they would not do while sober and are unable to judge accurately their ability to drive safely. Definite impairment of driving ability and memory is present. This level of intoxication is considered legally drunk in most states.	**.20%** At this level, a person is about 100 times more likely to cause a fatal accident if he or she drives. In a normal person, this BAC level is likely to cause a kind of amnesia known as an "alcohol blackout" in which the person cannot recall what happened while he or she was intoxicated.	**.60%** Most drinkers would be dead. Emergency rooms and police departments, however, recognize that a few drinkers with abnormally high tolerance do survive and even remain conscious at this level.

#3 Personal Risk

This section provides information about level of risk in four categories. "High risk" does not mean that you have (or will have) serious problems with alcohol. Neither does "low risk" mean that you won't have problems. But, *the higher your risk, the greater your chances of developing alcohol problems.*

DRINKING SEVERITY

Your severity: ____
Low (0–7)
Medium (8–15)
High (16–25)
Very High (26+)

This score indicates your level of risk based on the World Health Organization's AUDIT screening measure. The categories were developed by the National Institute on Alcohol Abuse and Alcoholism to advise drinkers entering treatment. Among college students, a score of 6 or more is an indicator of elevated risk.

TOLERANCE

Your tolerance level: ____
Low (0–60)
Medium (61–120)
High (121–180)
Very High (181+)

Peak monthly BAC is an estimate of alcohol tolerance. If you are reaching BAC levels beyond

the normal range (especially if you are not feeling much effect at lower BACs), you probably have a higher tolerance for alcohol. This might be partly hereditary and partly the result of changes in the body that occur with heavier drinking. People who have a higher tolerance are at greater risk for current and future alcohol problems. They also tend to experience fewer stimulating effects and greater depressant effects when drinking.

FAMILY RISK

Your family risk level: ____
Low (0–1)
Medium (2–3)
High (4–6)
Very High (7+)

People with a family history of alcohol problems are at greater risk themselves. The risk goes up more if the relatives are more numerous and/or more closely related. Those with a high family risk score *and* a high tolerance are at the greatest risk of all. If your scores place you at risk, you may want to seriously consider not drinking or consuming only small amounts of alcohol infrequently.

RISK TAKING AND ACCIDENTS

Has likely *driven* while impaired by alcohol? ____

Has likely *ridden with* an alcohol-impaired driver? ____

MYTH #1: Higher tolerance means you are not being harmed by alcohol.
Higher tolerance—the ability "to hold your liquor"—actually puts you at *greater* risk. The person with a high tolerance needs more alcohol to feel the same effects as those with lower tolerance. Not only is this financially expensive, but the high levels of toxins can significantly damage the body. Like a person who has no sense of pain, people with a high tolerance can damage their bodies without realizing it.

MYTH #2: Higher tolerance means that your body gets rid of alcohol at a faster rate than others.
Tolerance does not affect estimation of BAC. Tolerance refers to how people feel *at a given BAC*. Individuals do vary somewhat in their ability to process alcohol, but once alcohol is in the bloodstream, there is nothing that can be done to speed up the process of elimination. Fortunately, alcohol tolerance seems to be reversible with even brief periods of abstinence or reduced consumption. Some have found it helpful to set a moderate BAC limit (.06%, for instance) that they will not exceed for some period of time (2 months, for instance).

Alcohol, even at levels under the legal limit, decreases the ability to perceive and react to surroundings. If you reported driving after drinking three or more drinks (or have ridden with an intoxicated driver), you have greatly increased your risk for injuries or legal problems.

Excessive drinking is also related to unprotected sex (leading to an increased risk of sexually transmitted diseases (STDs)/HIV and pregnancy) and is a major factor in most cases of date rape. After drinking, people are also more likely to misjudge the actions of others as threatening and to react aggressively or violently.

Before you drink, consider a safe way to get home:

- Select a person you trust to be the designated driver for the night.
- Give your keys to a sober friend.
- Call a taxi—cab fare is cheaper than a DWI.
- Call a sober friend or family member and ask for a ride.

#4 The Norms

What percent of U.S. college students (same sex) drink more than you do?
  You said ____% Survey said ____%

What percent of U.S. college students do not drink at all in a typical week?
  You said ____% Survey said 32%

What percent of U.S. college students have two drinks or fewer in a typical week?
  You said ____% Survey said 51%

What percent of U.S. college students smoke marijuana at least once a year?
  You said ____% Survey said 25%

In addition to showing how your drinking fits in with national norms, this also shows how your estimates compared with actual survey responses. The drinking information is based on an anonymous survey of 38,331 U.S. undergraduates during 2003. The marijuana percent is drawn from a similar survey of 17,592 students. If your guesses were off, you're not alone! Several studies have shown that members of the campus community (including faculty and staff) tend to *overestimate* the number of students who drink heavily.

#5 Tobacco Use

Number of cigarettes per month ____
Number of years smoking ____

Most smokers are aware of the addictive nature of nicotine and the increased risk for disease. What people may *not* know is that the *combination* of tobacco and alcohol greatly increases the risk for oral, neck, and stomach cancers.

Those who choose to smoke should be aware of the impact of passive smoke on others. The toxic particles in tobacco smoke account for an estimated 53,000 deaths per year in the United States among nonsmokers—*more than the death rates for illegal drug use and murders combined!* Those concerned about the effects of secondhand smoke should limit their exposure to smoking and drinking environments.

#6 Resources

There are many local and national resources for students who want to explore their alcohol use further, including the following websites:

- www.factsontap.org (Alcohol and the college experience)
- www.collegedrinkingprevention.gov (Interactive learning about myths and facts of alcohol)
- www.alternativebreaks.org (Alcohol-free spring break programs)
- www.jointogether.org (News service, online discussion groups, and other alcohol-related resources)

Adapted from the work of W. R. Miller and colleagues at the Center on Alcoholism, Substance Abuse and Addictions, the University of New Mexico. For copyright information contact Scott Walters, UT School of Public Health, 5323 Harry Hines Blvd, V8.112, Dallas, TX 75390-9128.

165

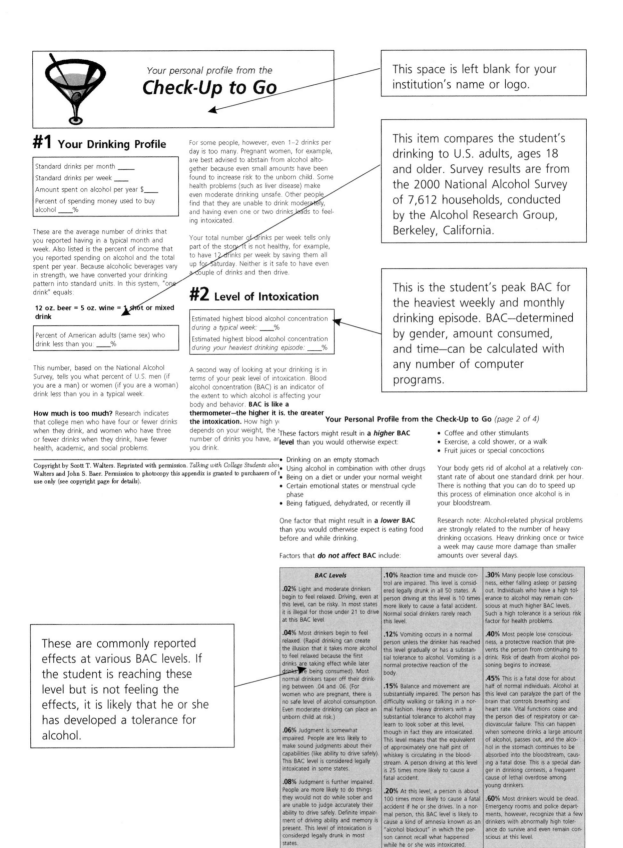

Your personal profile from the
Check-Up to Go

This space is left blank for your institution's name or logo.

#1 Your Drinking Profile

Standard drinks per month ____
Standard drinks per week ____
Amount spent on alcohol per year $____
Percent of spending money used to buy alcohol ____%

These are the average number of drinks that you reported having in a typical month and week. Also listed is the percent of income that you reported spending on alcohol and the total spent per year. Because alcoholic beverages vary in strength, we have converted your drinking pattern into standard units. In this system, "one drink" equals:

12 oz. beer = 5 oz. wine = 1 shot or mixed drink

Percent of American adults (same sex) who drink less than you: ____%

This number, based on the National Alcohol Survey, tells you what percent of U.S. men (if you are a man) or women (if you are a woman) drink less than you in a typical week.

How much is too much? Research indicates that college men who have four or fewer drinks when they drink, and women who have three or fewer drinks when they drink, have fewer health, academic, and social problems.

Copyright by Scott T. Walters. Reprinted with permission. *Talking with College Students about* Walters and John S. Baer. Permission to photocopy this appendix is granted to purchasers of l use only (see copyright page for details).

For some people, however, even 1–2 drinks per day is too many. Pregnant women, for example, are best advised to abstain from alcohol altogether because even small amounts have been found to increase risk to the unborn child. Some health problems (such as liver disease) make even moderate drinking unsafe. Other people find that they are unable to drink moderately, and having even one or two drinks leads to feeling intoxicated.

Your total number of drinks per week tells only part of the story. It is not healthy, for example, to have 12 drinks per week by saving them all up for Saturday. Neither is it safe to have even a couple of drinks and then drive.

#2 Level of Intoxication

Estimated highest blood alcohol concentration *during a typical week:* ____%
Estimated highest blood alcohol concentration *during your heaviest drinking episode:* ____%

A second way of looking at your drinking is in terms of your peak level of intoxication. Blood alcohol concentration (BAC) is an indicator of the extent to which alcohol is affecting your body and behavior. **BAC is like a thermometer—the higher it is, the greater the intoxication.** How high yo depends on your weight, the s number of drinks you have, ar you drink.

This item compares the student's drinking to U.S. adults, ages 18 and older. Survey results are from the 2000 National Alcohol Survey of 7,612 households, conducted by the Alcohol Research Group, Berkeley, California.

This is the student's peak BAC for the heaviest weekly and monthly drinking episode. BAC—determined by gender, amount consumed, and time—can be calculated with any number of computer programs.

These factors might result in **a higher BAC level** than you would otherwise expect:

- Drinking on an empty stomach
- Using alcohol in combination with other drugs
- Being on a diet or under your normal weight
- Certain emotional states or menstrual cycle phase
- Being fatigued, dehydrated, or recently ill

One factor that might result in a *lower* BAC than you would otherwise expect is eating food before and while drinking.

Factors that *do not affect* BAC include:

- Coffee and other stimulants
- Exercise, a cold shower, or a walk
- Fruit juices or special concoctions

Your body gets rid of alcohol at a relatively constant rate of about one standard drink per hour. There is nothing that you can do to speed up this process of elimination once alcohol is in your bloodstream.

Research note: Alcohol-related physical problems are strongly related to the number of heavy drinking occasions. Heavy drinking once or twice a week may cause more damage than smaller amounts over several days.

These are commonly reported effects at various BAC levels. If the student is reaching these level but is not feeling the effects, it is likely that he or she has developed a tolerance for alcohol.

BAC Levels		
.02% Light and moderate drinkers begin to feel relaxed. Driving, even at this level, can be risky. In most states it is illegal for those under 21 to drive at this BAC level.	**.10%** Reaction time and muscle control are impaired. This level is considered legally drunk in all 50 states. A person driving at this level is 10 times more likely to cause a fatal accident. Normal social drinkers rarely reach this level.	**.30%** Many people lose consciousness, either falling asleep or passing out. Individuals who have a high tolerance to alcohol may remain conscious at much higher BAC levels. Such a high tolerance is a serious risk factor for health problems.
.04% Most drinkers begin to feel relaxed. (Rapid drinking can create the illusion that it takes more alcohol to feel relaxed because the first drinks are taking effect while later drinks are being consumed). Most normal drinkers taper off their drinking between .04 and .06. (For women who are pregnant, there is no safe level of alcohol consumption. Even moderate drinking can place an unborn child at risk.)	**.12%** Vomiting occurs in a normal person unless the drinker has reached this level gradually or has a substantial tolerance to alcohol. Vomiting is a normal protective reaction of the body.	**.40%** Most people lose consciousness, a protective reaction that prevents the person from continuing to drink. Risk of death from alcohol poisoning begins to increase.
.06% Judgment is somewhat impaired. People are less likely to make sound judgments about their capabilities (like ability to drive safely). This BAC level is considered legally intoxicated in some states.	**.15%** Balance and movement are substantially impaired. The person has difficulty walking or talking in a normal fashion. Heavy drinkers with a substantial tolerance to alcohol may learn to look sober at this level, though in fact they are intoxicated. This level means that the equivalent of approximately one half pint of whiskey is circulating in the bloodstream. A person driving at this level is 25 times more likely to cause a fatal accident.	**.45%** This is a fatal dose for about half of normal individuals. Alcohol at this level can paralyze the part of the brain that controls breathing and heart rate. Vital functions cease and the person dies of respiratory or cardiovascular failure. This can happen when someone drinks a large amount of alcohol, passes out, and the alcohol in the stomach continues to be absorbed into the bloodstream, causing a fatal dose. This is a special danger in drinking contests, a frequent cause of lethal overdose among young drinkers.
.08% Judgment is further impaired. People are more likely to do things they would not do while sober and are unable to judge accurately their ability to drive safely. Definite impairment of driving ability and memory is present. This level of intoxication is considered legally drunk in most states.	**.20%** At this level, a person is about 100 times more likely to cause a fatal accident if he or she drives. In a normal person, this BAC level is likely to cause a kind of amnesia known as an "alcohol blackout" in which the person cannot recall what happened while he or she was intoxicated.	**.60%** Most drinkers would be dead. Emergency rooms and police departments, however, recognize that a few drinkers with abnormally high tolerance do survive and even remain conscious at this level.

#3 Personal Risk

This section provides information about level of risk in four categories. "High risk" does not mean that you have (or will have) serious problems with alcohol. Neither does "low risk" mean that you won't have problems. But, *the higher your risk, the greater your chances of developing alcohol problems.*

DRINKING SEVERITY

Your severity: ____
Low (0–7)
Medium (8–15)
High (16–25)
Very High (26+)

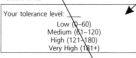

This score indicates your level of risk based on the World Health Organization's AUDIT screening measure. The categories were developed by the National Institute on Alcohol Abuse and Alcoholism to advise drinkers entering treatment. Among college students, a score of 6 or more is an indicator of elevated risk.

TOLERANCE

Your tolerance level: ____
Low (0–60)
Medium (61–120)
High (121–180)
Very High (181+)

Peak monthly BAC is an estimate of alcohol tolerance. If you are reaching BAC levels beyond

the normal range (especially if you are not feeling much effect at lower BACs), you probably have a higher tolerance for alcohol. This might be partly hereditary and partly the result of changes in the body that occur with heavier drinking. People who have a higher tolerance are at greater risk for current and future alcohol problems. They also tend to experience fewer stimulating effects and greater depressant effects when drinking.

FAMILY RISK

Your family risk level: ____
Low (0–1)
Medium (2–3)
High (4–6)
Very High (7+)

People with a family history of alcohol problems are at greater risk themselves. The risk goes up more if the relatives are more numerous and/or more closely related. Those with a high family risk score *and* a high tolerance are at the greatest risk of all. If your scores place you at risk, you may want to seriously consider not drinking or consuming only small amounts of alcohol infrequently.

RISK TAKING AND ACCIDENTS

Has likely *driven* while impaired by alcohol?
____

Has likely *ridden with* an alcohol-impaired driver? ____

MYTH #1: Higher tolerance means you are not being harmed by alcohol.
Higher tolerance—the ability "to hold your liquor"—actually puts you at *greater* risk. The person with a high tolerance needs more alcohol to [...] sive, but the high levels of t[...] people with a high tolerance [...]

MYTH #2: Higher tolerance [...]
Tolerance does not affect es[...] vary somewhat in their abilit[...] be done to speed up the pr[...] brief periods of abstinence c[...] (.06%, for instance) that the [...]

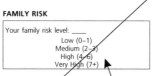

The severity/dependence score comes from the World Health Organization's Alcohol Use Disorders Identification Test (AUDIT), with permission from the author. Severity categories are those used in the NIAAA's Project MATCH study.

Tolerance and genetic risk questions come from the NIAAA's Project MATCH study. Tolerance is inferred from peak monthly BAC and is a risk factor for developing alcohol problems or alcohol dependence. Students who are reaching higher levels are likely not to be feeling the effects of alcohol to the same extent as a person with a lower tolerance. Tolerance level categories are those used in the NIAAA's Project MATCH study. More information on MATCH can be found at http://www.niaaa.nih.gov/press/1996/match-text.htm

Genetic risk score is determined by a weighted algorithm that takes into account the number of first- (1 point) and second- (2 points) degree relatives who are problem drinkers or alcoholics. The risk goes up more if the relatives are more numerous, the same gender, and/or more closely related to you. Those with a high family risk score *and* a high tolerance are at the greatest risk of all. Family risk categories are those used in the NIAAA's Project MATCH study.

[...] r Pers[...]
[...]els un[...]
[...] to pe[...]
[...]repo[...]
[...]rinks ([...]
[...]ou ha[...]
[...] or leg[...]

[...] also r[...]
[...]ncrease[...]
[...] (STDs[...]
[...]r in m[...]
[...]. After drinking, peop[...] to misjudge the actions of [...] and to react aggressively [...]

Before you drink, consider a[...]

- Select a person you trust to be the designated driver for the night.
- Give your keys to a sober friend.
- Call a taxi—cab fare is cheaper than a DWI.
- Call a sober friend or family member and ask for a ride.

#4 The Norms

What percent of U.S. college students (same sex) drink more than you do?
You said ____% Survey said ____%

What percent of U.S. college students do not drink at all in a typical week?
You said ____% Survey said 32%

What percent of U.S. college students have two drinks or fewer in a typical week?
You said ____% Survey said 51%

What percent of U.S. college students smoke marijuana at least once a year?
You said ____% Survey said 25%

In addition to showing how your drinking fits with national norms, this also shows how your estimates compared with actual survey responses. The drinking information is based on an anonymous survey of 38,331 U.S. undergradu-

College drinking norms are drawn from a sample of 38,331 U.S. undergraduate students who completed the 2003 Core Survey. All institutions used methods to ensure a random and representative sample of their respective student bodies. Marijuana norms were drawn from a similar national survey.

Listed are national information and referral sources. Colleges may wish to include local information or referral sources as well.

of nicotine and the increased risk for disease. What people may *not* know is that the *combination* of tobacco and alcohol greatly increases the risk for oral, neck, and stomach cancers.

Those who choose to smoke should be aware of the impact of passive smoke on others. The toxic particles in tobacco smoke account for an estimated 53,000 deaths per year in the United States among nonsmokers—*more than the death rates for illegal drug use and murders combined!* Those concerned about the effects of secondhand smoke should limit their exposure to smoking and drinking environments.

#6 Resources

There are many local and national resources for students who want to explore their alcohol use further, including the following websites:

- www.factsontap.org (Alcohol and the college experience)
- www.collegedrinkingprevention.gov (Interactive learning about myths and facts of alcohol)
- www.alternativebreaks.org (Alcohol-free spring break programs)
- www.jointogether.org (News service, online discussion groups, and other alcohol-related resources)

Adapted from the work of W. R. Miller and colleagues at the Center on Alcoholism, Substance Abuse and Addictions, the University of New Mexico. For copyright information contact Scott Walters, UT School of Public Health, 5323 Harry Hines Blvd, V8.112, Dallas, TX 75390-9128.

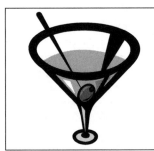

Coding Procedures for the
Check-Up to Go

#1 Your Drinking Profile

Standard drinks per month:
This amount is found by totaling the drinks per week in question 1, "For the past month, please describe a typical drinking week" and multiplying the amount by 4.3.

Standard drinks per week:
Direct from question 1.

Amount spent on alcohol per year:
Multiply the dollar amount in question 5, "How much would you estimate you spend on alcoholic beverages per week?" by 52.

Percent of income spent on alcohol:
Multiply the amount in question 11, "After school expenses, how much money do you have to spend in an average month?" by 12 to get an estimate of annual income. Divide the amount spent on alcohol per year by the annual income.

Percent of American adults (same sex) who drink less than you:
Compare the obtained drinks per week to the values in Chart 1, matching for sex. Write the percentile in the box. If student is not a drinker, write "NA" in the box and "34% of males also don't drink" or "44% of females also don't drink."

#2 Level of Intoxication

Highest BAC during a typical week:
From the weekly calendar, total the number of drinks consumed on the heaviest day. Taking into account weight, number of drinks, time, and gender, calculate a peak BAC for a typical week. (For an automatic calculation, download the BACCUS program at casaa.unm.edu or use a website such as www.progressive.com/RC/DSafety/rc_get_the_keys.asp) Write the number in the box.

Chart 1		
Drinks/week	%tile (Men)	%tile (Women)
0	34	44
1	61	79
2	65	83
3	72	89
4	75	90
5	76	91
6	79	93
7	81	94
8	82	94
9	83	95
10	84	95
11	87	96
12	88	97
13	89	97
14	89	98
15–17	90	98
18–19	91	99
20–23	92	99
24–26	93	99
27–30	94	99
31–36	95	99
37–42	96	99
43–49	97	99
50–59	98	99
60–69	98	> 99
70 and up	99	> 99

Highest BAC during your heaviest drinking episode:
Use the total number of drinks and hours indicated in question 2. Use the site above to calculate peak BAC for the past month. Write the number in the box. (We have used .45 as a maximum allowable BAC. If students exceed this, we also write, "This is a fatal dose" on the feedback.)

#3 Personal Risk Factors

DRINKING SEVERITY

Your severity:
Use the AUDIT (question 8) for this score. Questions a–h are scored 0, 1, 2, 3 or 4. Questions i–j are scored 0, 2, or 4 only. Total the amount and write this number in the severity box.

TOLERANCE

Your tolerance level:
This is the mg% form of the highest BAC over the last 30 days. Convert the BAC decimal amount into mg% amount by moving the decimal three places to the right. For instance, a decimal BAC of .06 equals a tolerance score of 60 (.12 converts to 120, .18 converts to 180, and so forth). Write the tolerance score in the box.

FAMILY RISK

Your family risk level:
Add the corresponding points for each blood relative indicated in question 3. Write the total in the family risk box.

Parents add 2 points for each positive
Brothers or sisters add 2 points for each positive
Grandparents add 1 point for each positive
Uncles or aunts add 1 point for each positive
First cousins add 1 point for each positive

169

Chart 2		
Drinks/week	% More (Males)	% More (Females)
0	72	65
1	64	52
2	58	43
3	54	37
4	51	33
5	45	26
6	42	23
7	40	21
8	38	18
9	37	17
10	30	11
11	29	11
12–13	26	9
14	25	8
15	21	5
16–17	20	5
18–19	19	5
20	14	3
21	13	3
22–23	13	2
24	12	2
25	9	2
26–29	9	1
30–34	6	1
35	5	1
36–39	4	<1
40–47	3	<1
48–49	2	<1
50–76	1	<1
77 and up	<1	<1

RISK TAKING AND ACCIDENTS

Has likely driven while impaired by alcohol:
For any answer other than 0, write "yes" next to *driven while impaired*.

Has likely ridden with an alcohol-impaired driver:
For any answer other than 0, write "yes" next to *ridden with an impaired driver*.

#4 The Norms

What percent of U.S. college students (same sex) drink more than you do?
Using drinks per week, compare this amount to Chart 2, matching for sex. Write the percent more in the box.

. . . U.S. college students . . . ?
For the last three questions, copy the answers directly from the CHUG assessment sheet.

#5 Tobacco Use

Number of cigarettes per month:
Multiply the number smoked per day by 30. Write the number in the box.

Number of years smoking:
Copy the number directly from the CHUG assessment sheet.

APPENDIX H

Values Cards

BRIEF DESCRIPTION

The Values Cards contain a list of 70 potentially important life values. They are formatted (10 per page) to be copied onto cardstock or preperforated business card paper.

TYPICAL APPLICATION

The Values Cards are used as part of an individual or group counseling session to help students identify deeply held values and weigh those in relation to their drinking. See Chapters 6 (p. 91) and 7 (p. 118).

ADMINISTRATIVE ISSUES

Time to administer: 10–20 minutes, with discussion
Time to score/interpret: n/a

COPYRIGHT ISSUES

Permission to copy? ☒ yes ☐ no
Contact: William R. Miller
                    Department of Psychology
                    University of New Mexico
                    Albuquerque, NM 87131

REFERENCES

Miller, W. R., & C'de Baca, J. (1994). Quantum change: Toward a psychology of transformation. In T. F. Heatherton & J. L. Weinberger (Eds.), *Can personality change?* (1st ed., pp. 253–280). Washington, DC: American Psychological Association.

Miller, W. R., & C'de Baca, J. (2001). *Quantum change: When epiphanies and sudden insights transform ordinary lives*. New York: Guilford Press.

ACCEPTANCE to be accepted as I am	**AUTHORITY** to be in charge of others
ACCURACY to be correct in my opinions and actions	**AUTONOMY** to be self-determining and independent
ACHIEVEMENT to accomplish and achieve	**BEAUTY** to appreciate beauty around me
ADVENTURE to have new and exciting experiences	**CARING** to take care of others
ATTRACTIVENESS to be physically attractive	**COMFORT** to have a pleasant, enjoyable life

COMMITMENT to make a long-lasting and deep commitment to another person	CREATIVITY to have new and original ideas
COMPASSION to feel and show concern for others	DEPENDABILITY to be reliable and trustworthy
COMPLEXITY to have a life full of variety and change	DUTY to carry out my duties and responsibilities
CONTRIBUTION to make a contribution that will last after I am gone	ECOLOGY to live in harmony with and protect the environment
COURTESY to be polite and considerate to others	FAME to be known and recognized

FAMILY to have a happy, loving family	GENEROSITY to give what I have to others
FLEXIBILITY to adjust to new or unusual situations easily	GENUINENESS to behave in a manner that is true to who I am
FORGIVENESS to be forgiving of others	GOD'S WILL to seek and obey the will of God
FRIENDS to have close, supportive friends	GROWTH to keep changing and growing
FUN to play and have fun	HEALTH to be physically well and healthy

HELPFULNESS to be helpful to others	**INDUSTRY** to work hard and well at my life tasks
HONESTY to be truthful and genuine	**INNER PEACE** to experience personal peace
HUMILITY to be modest and unassuming	**INTIMACY** to share my innermost experience with others
HUMOR to see the humorous side of myself and the world	**JUSTICE** to promote equal and fair treatment for all
INDEPENDENCE to be free from dependence on others	**KNOWLEDGE** to learn and possess valuable knowledge

LEISURE to take time to relax and enjoy	**MODERATION** to avoid excesses and find a middle ground
LOGIC to live rationally and sensibly	**MONOGAMY** to have one close, loving relationship
LOVED to be loved by those close to me	**ORDERLINESS** to have a life that is well-ordered and organized
LOVING to give love to others	**PLEASURE** to have experiences that feel good
MASTERY to be competent in my everyday activities	**POPULARITY** to be well-liked by many people

POWER to have control over others	ROMANCE to have intense, exciting love in my life
PURPOSE to have meaning and direction in my life	SAFETY to be safe and secure
REALISM to see and act realistically and practically	SELF-ACCEPTANCE to like myself as I am
RESPONSIBILITY to make and carry out important decisions	SELF-CONTROL to be self-disciplined and govern my own activities
RISK to take risks and chances	SELF-ESTEEM to feel positive about myself

SELF-KNOWLEDGE to have a deep, honest understanding of myself	STABILITY to have a life that stays fairly consistent
SERVICE to be of service to others	STRENGTH to be physically strong
SEXUALITY to have an active and satisfying sex life	TOLERANCE to accept and respect those different from me
SIMPLICITY to live life simply, with minimal needs	VIRTUE to live a morally pure and excellent life
SPIRITUALITY to grow spiritually	WEALTH to have plenty of money

APPENDIX I

Self–Monitoring Cards

BRIEF DESCRIPTION

The Self-Monitoring Cards provide a way for students to keep track of their drinking over a period of time.

TYPICAL APPLICATION

The Self-Monitoring Cards are used as part of a counseling session to structure a discussion about how much, how often, and with whom a student is drinking. They can also be used to set goals or monitor drinking changes over time. See Chapter 6 (p. 93).

ADMINISTRATIVE ISSUES

Time to administer: 3–5 minutes, for instruction
Time to score/interpret: variable
Computerized scoring available?   ☐ yes   ☒ no
College student norms available?   ☒ yes   ☐ no

COPYRIGHT ISSUES

Permission to copy?   ☒ yes   ☐ no

REFERENCES

Baer, J. S., Marlatt, G. A., Kivlahan, D. R., Fromme, K., Larimer, M., & Williams, E. (1992). An experimental test of three methods of alcohol risk reduction with young adults. *Journal of Consulting and Clinical Psychology, 60*(6), 974–979.

Dimeff, L. A., Baer, J. S., Kivlahan, D. R., & Marlatt, G. A. (1999). *Brief alcohol screening and intervention for college students: A harm reduction approach.* New York: Guilford Press.

Larimer, M. E., Turner, A. P., Anderson, B. K., Fader, J. S., Kilmer, J. R., Palmer, R. S., & Cronce, J. M. (2001). Evaluating a brief alcohol intervention with fraternities. *Journal of Studies on Alcohol, 62*(3), 370–380.

BAC Self-Monitoring Card

Date	Start time	End time	Number of drinks			Total no. of drinks	Situation
			Beer	Wine	Liquor		

Date	Start time	End time	Number of drinks			Total no. of drinks	Situation
			Beer	Wine	Liquor		

A standard drink is approximately 12 ounces of beer, 4 ounces of wine, or 1¼ ounces of 80-proof spirits.

APPENDIX J

BAC Cards

BRIEF DESCRIPTION

The BAC cards give an estimated blood alcohol concentration (BAC), based on the gender of the student, rate of drinking, and time spent drinking.

TYPICAL APPLICATION

The BAC cards are used to help students monitor the amount of alcohol in their bloodstream. See Chapter 6 (p. 93).

ADMINISTRATIVE ISSUES

Time to administer: 3–5 minutes, for instruction
Time to score/interpret: n/a

COPYRIGHT ISSUES

Permission to copy?   ☒ yes   ☐ no
Laminated, gender- and weight-specific cards are available at www.baczone.biz
A free BAC calculation program is available at casaa.unm.edu/dload.html

REFERENCES

See www.baczone.biz.
See www.factsontap.org.
See getfit.samhsa.gov/Alcohol/Tests/bac.aspx.

BAC Cards for Males (page 1 of 4)

BACs for 120-pound male

No. of drinks	Hours										
	0	1	2	3	4	5	6	7	8	9	10
1	.031	.015	0	0	0	0	0	0	0	0	0
2	.062	.046	.030	.014	0	0	0	0	0	0	0
3	.094	.078	.062	.046	.030	.014	0	0	0	0	0
4	.125	.109	.093	.077	.061	.045	.029	.013	0	0	0
5	.156	.140	.124	.108	.092	.076	.060	.044	.028	.012	0
6	.188	.172	.156	.140	.124	.108	.092	.076	.060	.044	.028
7	.219	.203	.187	.171	.155	.139	.123	.107	.091	.075	.059
8	.250	.234	.218	.202	.186	.170	.154	.138	.122	.106	.090
9	.281	.265	.249	.233	.217	.201	.185	.169	.153	.137	.121
10	.312	.296	.280	.264	.248	.232	.216	.200	.184	.168	.152
11	.344	.328	.312	.296	.280	.264	.248	.232	.216	.200	.184
12	.375	.359	.343	.327	.311	.295	.279	.263	.247	.231	.215
13	.406	.390	.374	.358	.342	.326	.310	.294	.278	.262	.246
14	.438	.422	.406	.390	.374	.358	.342	.326	.310	.294	.278
15	.469	.453	.437	.421	.405	.389	.373	.357	.341	.325	.309

BACs for 130-pound male

No. of drinks	Hours										
	0	1	2	3	4	5	6	7	8	9	10
1	.029	.013	0	0	0	0	0	0	0	0	0
2	.058	.042	.026	.010	0	0	0	0	0	0	0
3	.087	.071	.055	.039	.023	.007	0	0	0	0	0
4	.115	.099	.083	.067	.051	.035	.019	.003	0	0	0
5	.144	.128	.112	.096	.080	.064	.048	.032	.016	0	0
6	.173	.157	.141	.125	.109	.093	.077	.061	.045	.029	.013
7	.202	.186	.170	.154	.138	.122	.106	.090	.074	.058	.042
8	.231	.215	.199	.183	.167	.151	.135	.119	.103	.087	.071
9	.260	.244	.228	.212	.196	.180	.164	.148	.132	.116	.100
10	.288	.272	.256	.240	.224	.208	.192	.176	.160	.144	.128
11	.317	.301	.285	.269	.253	.237	.221	.205	.189	.173	.157
12	.346	.330	.314	.298	.282	.266	.250	.234	.218	.202	.186
13	.375	.359	.343	.327	.311	.295	.279	.263	.247	.231	.215
14	.404	.388	.372	.356	.340	.324	.308	.292	.276	.260	.244
15	.433	.417	.401	.385	.369	.353	.337	.321	.305	.289	.273

BACs for 140-pound male

No. of drinks	Hours										
	0	1	2	3	4	5	6	7	8	9	10
1	.027	.011	0	0	0	0	0	0	0	0	0
2	.054	.038	.022	.006	0	0	0	0	0	0	0
3	.080	.064	.048	.032	.016	0	0	0	0	0	0
4	.107	.091	.075	.059	.043	.027	.011	0	0	0	0
5	.134	.118	.102	.086	.070	.054	.038	.022	.006	0	0
6	.161	.145	.129	.113	.097	.081	.065	.049	.033	.017	.001
7	.188	.172	.156	.140	.124	.108	.092	.076	.060	.044	.028
8	.214	.198	.182	.166	.150	.134	.118	.102	.086	.070	.054
9	.241	.225	.209	.193	.177	.161	.145	.129	.113	.097	.081
10	.268	.252	.236	.220	.204	.188	.172	.156	.140	.124	.108
11	.295	.279	.263	.247	.231	.215	.199	.183	.167	.151	.135
12	.321	.305	.289	.273	.257	.241	.225	.209	.193	.177	.161
13	.348	.332	.316	.300	.284	.268	.252	.236	.220	.204	.188
14	.375	.359	.343	.327	.311	.295	.279	.263	.247	.231	.215
15	.402	.386	.370	.354	.338	.322	.306	.290	.274	.258	.242

BACs for 150-pound male

No. of drinks	Hours										
	0	1	2	3	4	5	6	7	8	9	10
1	.025	.009	0	0	0	0	0	0	0	0	0
2	.050	.034	.018	.002	0	0	0	0	0	0	0
3	.075	.059	.043	.027	.011	0	0	0	0	0	0
4	.100	.084	.068	.052	.036	.020	.004	0	0	0	0
5	.125	.109	.093	.077	.061	.045	.029	.013	0	0	0
6	.150	.134	.118	.102	.086	.070	.054	.038	.022	.006	0
7	.175	.159	.143	.127	.111	.095	.079	.063	.047	.031	.015
8	.200	.184	.168	.152	.136	.120	.104	.088	.072	.056	.040
9	.225	.209	.193	.177	.161	.145	.129	.113	.097	.081	.065
10	.250	.234	.218	.202	.186	.170	.154	.138	.122	.106	.090
11	.275	.259	.243	.227	.211	.195	.179	.163	.147	.131	.115
12	.300	.284	.268	.252	.236	.220	.204	.188	.172	.156	.140
13	.325	.309	.293	.277	.261	.245	.229	.213	.197	.181	.165
14	.350	.334	.318	.302	.286	.270	.254	.238	.222	.206	.190
15	.375	.359	.343	.327	.311	.295	.279	.263	.247	.231	.215

BAC Cards for Males (page 2 of 4)

BACs for 160-pound male

No. of drinks	0	1	2	3	4	5	6	7	8	9	10
						Hours					
1	.023	.007	0	0	0	0	0	0	0	0	0
2	.047	.031	.015	0	0	0	0	0	0	0	0
3	.070	.054	.038	.022	.006	0	0	0	0	0	0
4	.094	.078	.062	.046	.030	.014	0	0	0	0	0
5	.117	.101	.085	.069	.053	.037	.021	.005	0	0	0
6	.141	.125	.109	.093	.077	.061	.045	.029	.013	0	0
7	.164	.148	.132	.116	.100	.084	.068	.052	.036	.020	.004
8	.188	.172	.156	.140	.124	.108	.092	.076	.060	.044	.028
9	.211	.195	.179	.163	.147	.131	.115	.099	.083	.067	.051
10	.234	.218	.202	.186	.170	.154	.138	.122	.106	.090	.074
11	.258	.242	.226	.210	.194	.178	.162	.146	.130	.114	.098
12	.281	.265	.249	.233	.217	.201	.185	.169	.153	.137	.121
13	.305	.289	.273	.257	.241	.225	.209	.193	.177	.161	.145
14	.328	.312	.296	.280	.264	.248	.232	.216	.200	.184	.168
15	.352	.336	.320	.304	.288	.272	.256	.240	.224	.208	.192

BACs for 170-pound male

No. of drinks	0	1	2	3	4	5	6	7	8	9	10
						Hours					
1	.022	.006	0	0	0	0	0	0	0	0	0
2	.044	.028	.012	0	0	0	0	0	0	0	0
3	.066	.050	.034	.018	.002	0	0	0	0	0	0
4	.088	.072	.056	.040	.024	.008	0	0	0	0	0
5	.110	.094	.078	.062	.046	.030	.014	0	0	0	0
6	.132	.116	.100	.084	.068	.052	.036	.020	.004	0	0
7	.154	.138	.122	.106	.090	.074	.058	.042	.026	.010	0
8	.176	.160	.144	.128	.112	.096	.080	.064	.048	.032	.016
9	.199	.183	.167	.151	.135	.119	.103	.087	.071	.055	.039
10	.221	.205	.189	.173	.157	.141	.125	.109	.093	.077	.061
11	.243	.227	.211	.195	.179	.163	.147	.131	.115	.099	.083
12	.265	.249	.233	.217	.201	.185	.169	.153	.137	.121	.105
13	.287	.271	.255	.239	.223	.207	.191	.175	.159	.143	.127
14	.309	.293	.277	.261	.245	.229	.213	.197	.181	.165	.149
15	.331	.315	.299	.283	.267	.251	.235	.219	.203	.187	.171

BACs for 180-pound male

No. of drinks	0	1	2	3	4	5	6	7	8	9	10
						Hours					
1	.021	.005	0	0	0	0	0	0	0	0	0
2	.042	.026	.010	0	0	0	0	0	0	0	0
3	.062	.046	.030	.014	0	0	0	0	0	0	0
4	.083	.067	.051	.035	.019	.003	0	0	0	0	0
5	.104	.088	.072	.056	.040	.024	.008	0	0	0	0
6	.125	.109	.093	.077	.061	.045	.029	.013	0	0	0
7	.146	.130	.114	.098	.082	.066	.050	.034	.018	.002	0
8	.167	.151	.135	.119	.103	.087	.071	.055	.039	.023	.007
9	.188	.172	.156	.140	.124	.108	.092	.076	.060	.044	.028
10	.208	.192	.176	.160	.144	.128	.112	.096	.080	.064	.048
11	.229	.213	.197	.181	.165	.149	.133	.117	.101	.085	.069
12	.250	.234	.218	.202	.186	.170	.154	.138	.122	.106	.090
13	.271	.255	.239	.223	.207	.191	.175	.159	.143	.127	.111
14	.292	.276	.260	.244	.228	.212	.196	.180	.164	.148	.132
15	.312	.296	.280	.264	.248	.232	.216	.200	.184	.168	.152

BACs for 190-pound male

No. of drinks	0	1	2	3	4	5	6	7	8	9	10
						Hours					
1	.020	.004	0	0	0	0	0	0	0	0	0
2	.039	.023	.007	0	0	0	0	0	0	0	0
3	.059	.043	.027	.011	0	0	0	0	0	0	0
4	.079	.063	.047	.031	.015	0	0	0	0	0	0
5	.099	.083	.067	.051	.035	.019	.003	0	0	0	0
6	.118	.102	.086	.070	.054	.038	.022	.006	0	0	0
7	.138	.122	.106	.090	.074	.058	.042	.026	.010	0	0
8	.158	.142	.126	.110	.094	.078	.062	.046	.030	.014	0
9	.178	.162	.146	.130	.114	.098	.082	.066	.050	.034	.018
10	.197	.181	.165	.149	.133	.117	.101	.085	.069	.053	.037
11	.217	.201	.185	.169	.153	.137	.121	.105	.089	.073	.057
12	.237	.221	.205	.189	.173	.157	.141	.125	.109	.093	.077
13	.257	.241	.225	.209	.193	.177	.161	.145	.129	.113	.097
14	.276	.260	.244	.228	.212	.196	.180	.164	.148	.132	.116
15	.296	.280	.264	.248	.232	.216	.200	.184	.168	.152	.136

BAC Cards for Males (page 3 of 4)

BACs for 200-pound male

No. of drinks	0	1	2	3	4	5	6	7	8	9	10
1	.019	.003	0	0	0	0	0	0	0	0	0
2	.038	.022	.006	0	0	0	0	0	0	0	0
3	.056	.040	.024	.008	0	0	0	0	0	0	0
4	.075	.059	.043	.027	.011	0	0	0	0	0	0
5	.094	.078	.062	.046	.030	.014	0	0	0	0	0
6	.113	.097	.081	.065	.049	.033	.017	.001	0	0	0
7	.131	.115	.099	.083	.067	.051	.035	.019	.003	0	0
8	.150	.134	.118	.102	.086	.070	.054	.038	.022	.006	0
9	.169	.153	.137	.121	.105	.089	.073	.057	.041	.025	.009
10	.188	.172	.156	.140	.124	.108	.092	.076	.060	.044	.028
11	.206	.190	.174	.158	.142	.126	.110	.094	.078	.062	.046
12	.225	.209	.193	.177	.161	.145	.129	.113	.097	.081	.065
13	.244	.228	.212	.196	.180	.164	.148	.132	.116	.100	.084
14	.263	.247	.231	.215	.199	.183	.167	.151	.135	.119	.103
15	.281	.265	.249	.233	.217	.201	.185	.169	.153	.137	.121

Hours

BACs for 210-pound male

No. of drinks	0	1	2	3	4	5	6	7	8	9	10
1	.018	.002	0	0	0	0	0	0	0	0	0
2	.036	.020	.004	0	0	0	0	0	0	0	0
3	.054	.038	.022	.006	0	0	0	0	0	0	0
4	.071	.055	.039	.023	.007	0	0	0	0	0	0
5	.089	.073	.057	.041	.025	.009	0	0	0	0	0
6	.107	.091	.075	.059	.043	.027	.011	0	0	0	0
7	.125	.109	.093	.077	.061	.045	.029	.013	0	0	0
8	.143	.127	.111	.095	.079	.063	.047	.031	.015	0	0
9	.161	.145	.129	.113	.097	.081	.065	.049	.033	.017	.001
10	.179	.163	.147	.131	.115	.099	.083	.067	.051	.035	.019
11	.196	.180	.164	.148	.132	.116	.100	.084	.068	.052	.036
12	.214	.198	.182	.166	.150	.134	.118	.102	.086	.070	.054
13	.232	.216	.200	.184	.168	.152	.136	.120	.104	.088	.072
14	.250	.234	.218	.202	.186	.170	.154	.138	.122	.106	.090
15	.268	.252	.236	.220	.204	.188	.172	.156	.140	.124	.108

Hours

BACs for 220-pound male

No. of drinks	0	1	2	3	4	5	6	7	8	9	10
1	.017	.001	0	0	0	0	0	0	0	0	0
2	.034	.018	.002	0	0	0	0	0	0	0	0
3	.051	.035	.019	.003	0	0	0	0	0	0	0
4	.068	.052	.036	.020	.004	0	0	0	0	0	0
5	.085	.069	.053	.037	.021	.005	0	0	0	0	0
6	.102	.086	.070	.054	.038	.022	.006	0	0	0	0
7	.119	.103	.087	.071	.055	.039	.023	.007	0	0	0
8	.136	.120	.104	.088	.072	.056	.040	.024	.008	0	0
9	.153	.137	.121	.105	.089	.073	.057	.041	.025	.009	0
10	.170	.154	.138	.122	.106	.090	.074	.058	.042	.026	.010
11	.188	.172	.156	.140	.124	.108	.092	.076	.060	.044	.028
12	.205	.189	.173	.157	.141	.125	.109	.093	.077	.061	.045
13	.222	.206	.190	.174	.158	.142	.126	.110	.094	.078	.062
14	.239	.223	.207	.191	.175	.159	.143	.127	.111	.095	.079
15	.256	.240	.224	.208	.192	.176	.160	.144	.128	.112	.096

Hours

BACs for 230-pound male

No. of drinks	0	1	2	3	4	5	6	7	8	9	10
1	.016	0	0	0	0	0	0	0	0	0	0
2	.033	.017	.001	0	0	0	0	0	0	0	0
3	.049	.033	.017	.001	0	0	0	0	0	0	0
4	.065	.049	.033	.017	.001	0	0	0	0	0	0
5	.082	.066	.050	.034	.018	.002	0	0	0	0	0
6	.098	.082	.066	.050	.034	.018	.002	0	0	0	0
7	.114	.098	.082	.066	.050	.034	.018	.002	0	0	0
8	.130	.114	.098	.082	.066	.050	.034	.018	.002	0	0
9	.147	.131	.115	.099	.083	.067	.051	.035	.019	.003	0
10	.163	.147	.131	.115	.099	.083	.067	.051	.035	.019	.003
11	.179	.163	.147	.131	.115	.099	.083	.067	.051	.035	.019
12	.196	.180	.164	.148	.132	.116	.100	.084	.068	.052	.036
13	.212	.196	.180	.164	.148	.132	.116	.100	.084	.068	.052
14	.228	.212	.196	.180	.164	.148	.132	.116	.100	.084	.068
15	.245	.229	.213	.197	.181	.165	.149	.133	.117	.101	.085

Hours

BAC Cards for Males (page 4 of 4)

BACs for 240-pound male

No. of drinks	0	1	2	3	4	Hours 5	6	7	8	9	10
1	.016	0	0	0	0	0	0	0	0	0	0
2	.031	.015	0	0	0	0	0	0	0	0	0
3	.047	.031	.015	0	0	0	0	0	0	0	0
4	.062	.046	.030	.014	0	0	0	0	0	0	0
5	.078	.062	.046	.030	.014	0	0	0	0	0	0
6	.094	.078	.062	.046	.030	.014	0	0	0	0	0
7	.109	.093	.077	.061	.045	.029	.013	0	0	0	0
8	.125	.109	.093	.077	.061	.045	.029	.013	0	0	0
9	.141	.125	.109	.093	.077	.061	.045	.029	.013	0	0
10	.156	.140	.124	.108	.092	.076	.060	.044	.028	.012	0
11	.172	.156	.140	.124	.108	.092	.076	.060	.044	.028	.012
12	.188	.172	.156	.140	.124	.108	.092	.076	.060	.044	.028
13	.203	.187	.171	.155	.139	.123	.107	.091	.075	.059	.043
14	.219	.203	.187	.171	.155	.139	.123	.107	.091	.075	.059
15	.234	.218	.202	.186	.170	.154	.138	.122	.106	.090	.074

BACs for 250-pound male

No. of drinks	0	1	2	3	4	Hours 5	6	7	8	9	10
1	.015	0	0	0	0	0	0	0	0	0	0
2	.030	.014	0	0	0	0	0	0	0	0	0
3	.045	.029	.013	0	0	0	0	0	0	0	0
4	.060	.044	.028	.012	0	0	0	0	0	0	0
5	.075	.059	.043	.027	.011	0	0	0	0	0	0
6	.090	.074	.058	.042	.026	.010	0	0	0	0	0
7	.105	.089	.073	.057	.041	.025	.009	0	0	0	0
8	.120	.104	.088	.072	.056	.040	.024	.008	0	0	0
9	.135	.119	.103	.087	.071	.055	.039	.023	.007	0	0
10	.150	.134	.118	.102	.086	.070	.054	.038	.022	.006	0
11	.165	.149	.133	.117	.101	.085	.069	.053	.037	.021	.005
12	.180	.164	.148	.132	.116	.100	.084	.068	.052	.036	.020
13	.195	.179	.163	.147	.131	.115	.099	.083	.067	.051	.035
14	.210	.194	.178	.162	.146	.130	.114	.098	.082	.066	.050
15	.225	.209	.193	.177	.161	.145	.129	.113	.097	.081	.065

BACs for 260-pound male

No. of drinks	0	1	2	3	4	Hours 5	6	7	8	9	10
1	.014	0	0	0	0	0	0	0	0	0	0
2	.029	.013	0	0	0	0	0	0	0	0	0
3	.043	.027	.011	0	0	0	0	0	0	0	0
4	.058	.042	.026	.010	0	0	0	0	0	0	0
5	.072	.056	.040	.024	.008	0	0	0	0	0	0
6	.087	.071	.055	.039	.023	.007	0	0	0	0	0
7	.101	.085	.069	.053	.037	.021	.005	0	0	0	0
8	.115	.099	.083	.067	.051	.035	.019	.003	0	0	0
9	.130	.114	.098	.082	.066	.050	.034	.018	.002	0	0
10	.144	.128	.112	.096	.080	.064	.048	.032	.016	0	0
11	.159	.143	.127	.111	.095	.079	.063	.047	.031	.015	0
12	.173	.157	.141	.125	.109	.093	.077	.061	.045	.029	.013
13	.188	.172	.156	.140	.124	.108	.092	.076	.060	.044	.028
14	.202	.186	.170	.154	.138	.122	.106	.090	.074	.058	.042
15	.216	.200	.184	.168	.152	.136	.120	.104	.088	.072	.056

BACs for 270-pound male

No. of drinks	0	1	2	3	4	Hours 5	6	7	8	9	10
1	.014	0	0	0	0	0	0	0	0	0	0
2	.028	.012	0	0	0	0	0	0	0	0	0
3	.042	.026	.010	0	0	0	0	0	0	0	0
4	.056	.040	.024	.008	0	0	0	0	0	0	0
5	.069	.053	.037	.021	.005	0	0	0	0	0	0
6	.083	.067	.051	.035	.019	.003	0	0	0	0	0
7	.097	.081	.065	.049	.033	.017	.001	0	0	0	0
8	.111	.095	.079	.063	.047	.031	.015	0	0	0	0
9	.125	.109	.093	.077	.061	.045	.029	.013	0	0	0
10	.139	.123	.107	.091	.075	.059	.043	.027	.011	0	0
11	.153	.137	.121	.105	.089	.073	.057	.041	.025	.009	0
12	.167	.151	.135	.119	.103	.087	.071	.055	.039	.023	.007
13	.181	.165	.149	.133	.117	.101	.085	.069	.053	.037	.021
14	.194	.178	.162	.146	.130	.114	.098	.082	.066	.050	.034
15	.208	.192	.176	.160	.144	.128	.112	.096	.080	.064	.048

BAC Cards for Females (page 1 of 4)

BACs for 100-pound female

No. of drinks	Hours										
	0	1	2	3	4	5	6	7	8	9	10
1	.045	.029	.013	0	0	0	0	0	0	0	0
2	.090	.074	.058	.042	.026	.010	0	0	0	0	0
3	.135	.119	.103	.087	.071	.055	.039	.023	.007	0	0
4	.180	.164	.148	.132	.116	.100	.084	.068	.052	.036	.020
5	.225	.209	.193	.177	.161	.145	.129	.113	.097	.081	.065
6	.270	.254	.238	.222	.206	.190	.174	.158	.142	.126	.110
7	.315	.299	.283	.267	.251	.235	.219	.203	.187	.171	.155
8	.360	.344	.328	.312	.296	.280	.264	.248	.232	.216	.200
9	.405	.389	.373	.357	.341	.325	.309	.293	.277	.261	.245
10	.450	.434	.418	.402	.386	.370	.354	.338	.322	.306	.290
11	.495	.479	.463	.447	.431	.415	.399	.383	.367	.351	.335
12	.540	.524	.508	.492	.476	.460	.444	.428	.412	.396	.380
13	.585	.569	.553	.537	.521	.505	.489	.473	.457	.441	.425
14	***	***	.598	.582	.566	.550	.534	.518	.502	.486	.470
15	***	***	***	***	***	.595	.579	.563	.547	.531	.515

BACs for 110-pound female

No. of drinks	Hours										
	0	1	2	3	4	5	6	7	8	9	10
1	.041	.025	.009	0	0	0	0	0	0	0	0
2	.082	.066	.050	.034	.018	.002	0	0	0	0	0
3	.123	.107	.091	.075	.059	.043	.027	.011	0	0	0
4	.164	.148	.132	.116	.100	.084	.068	.052	.036	.020	.004
5	.205	.189	.173	.157	.141	.125	.109	.093	.077	.061	.045
6	.245	.229	.213	.197	.181	.165	.149	.133	.117	.101	.085
7	.286	.270	.254	.238	.222	.206	.190	.174	.158	.142	.126
8	.327	.311	.295	.279	.263	.247	.231	.215	.199	.183	.167
9	.368	.352	.336	.320	.304	.288	.272	.256	.240	.224	.208
10	.409	.393	.377	.361	.345	.329	.313	.297	.281	.265	.249
11	.450	.434	.418	.402	.386	.370	.354	.338	.322	.306	.290
12	.491	.475	.459	.443	.427	.411	.395	.379	.363	.347	.331
13	.532	.516	.500	.484	.468	.452	.436	.420	.404	.388	.372
14	.573	.557	.541	.525	.509	.493	.477	.461	.445	.429	.413
15	***	.598	.582	.566	.550	.534	.518	.502	.486	.470	.454

BACs for 120-pound female

No. of drinks	Hours										
	0	1	2	3	4	5	6	7	8	9	10
1	.038	.022	.006	0	0	0	0	0	0	0	0
2	.075	.059	.043	.027	.011	0	0	0	0	0	0
3	.113	.097	.081	.065	.049	.033	.017	.001	0	0	0
4	.150	.134	.118	.102	.086	.070	.054	.038	.022	.006	0
5	.188	.172	.156	.140	.124	.108	.092	.076	.060	.044	.028
6	.225	.209	.193	.177	.161	.145	.129	.113	.097	.081	.065
7	.263	.247	.231	.215	.199	.183	.167	.151	.135	.119	.103
8	.300	.284	.268	.252	.236	.220	.204	.188	.172	.156	.140
9	.338	.322	.306	.290	.274	.258	.242	.226	.210	.194	.178
10	.375	.359	.343	.327	.311	.295	.279	.263	.247	.231	.215
11	.413	.397	.381	.365	.349	.333	.317	.301	.285	.269	.253
12	.450	.434	.418	.402	.386	.370	.354	.338	.322	.306	.290
13	.488	.472	.456	.440	.424	.408	.392	.376	.360	.344	.328
14	.525	.509	.493	.477	.461	.445	.429	.413	.397	.381	.365
15	.562	.546	.530	.514	.498	.482	.466	.450	.434	.418	.402

BACs for 130-pound female

No. of drinks	Hours										
	0	1	2	3	4	5	6	7	8	9	10
1	.035	.019	.003	0	0	0	0	0	0	0	0
2	.069	.053	.037	.021	.005	0	0	0	0	0	0
3	.104	.088	.072	.056	.040	.024	.008	0	0	0	0
4	.138	.122	.106	.090	.074	.058	.042	.026	.010	0	0
5	.173	.157	.141	.125	.109	.093	.077	.061	.045	.029	.013
6	.208	.192	.176	.160	.144	.128	.112	.096	.080	.064	.048
7	.242	.226	.210	.194	.178	.162	.146	.130	.114	.098	.082
8	.277	.261	.245	.229	.213	.197	.181	.165	.149	.133	.117
9	.312	.296	.280	.264	.248	.232	.216	.200	.184	.168	.152
10	.346	.330	.314	.298	.282	.266	.250	.234	.218	.202	.186
11	.381	.365	.349	.333	.317	.301	.285	.269	.253	.237	.221
12	.415	.399	.383	.367	.351	.335	.319	.303	.287	.271	.255
13	.450	.434	.418	.402	.386	.370	.354	.338	.322	.306	.290
14	.485	.469	.453	.437	.421	.405	.389	.373	.357	.341	.325
15	.519	.503	.487	.471	.455	.439	.423	.407	.391	.375	.359

BAC Cards for Females *(page 2 of 4)*

BACs for 140-pound female

No. of drinks	0	1	2	3	4	5	6	7	8	9	10
						Hours					
1	.032	.016	0	0	0	0	0	0	0	0	0
2	.064	.048	.032	.016	0	0	0	0	0	0	0
3	.096	.080	.064	.048	.032	.016	0	0	0	0	0
4	.129	.113	.097	.081	.065	.049	.033	.017	.001	0	0
5	.161	.145	.129	.113	.097	.081	.065	.049	.033	.017	.001
6	.193	.177	.161	.145	.129	.113	.097	.081	.065	.049	.033
7	.225	.209	.193	.177	.161	.145	.129	.113	.097	.081	.065
8	.257	.241	.225	.209	.193	.177	.161	.145	.129	.113	.097
9	.289	.273	.257	.241	.225	.209	.193	.177	.161	.145	.129
10	.321	.305	.289	.273	.257	.241	.225	.209	.193	.177	.161
11	.354	.338	.322	.306	.290	.274	.258	.242	.226	.210	.194
12	.386	.370	.354	.338	.322	.306	.290	.274	.258	.242	.226
13	.418	.402	.386	.370	.354	.338	.322	.306	.290	.274	.258
14	.450	.434	.418	.402	.386	.370	.354	.338	.322	.306	.290
15	.482	.466	.450	.434	.418	.402	.386	.370	.354	.338	.322

BACs for 150-pound female

No. of drinks	0	1	2	3	4	5	6	7	8	9	10
						Hours					
1	.030	.014	0	0	0	0	0	0	0	0	0
2	.060	.044	.028	.012	0	0	0	0	0	0	0
3	.090	.074	.058	.042	.026	.010	0	0	0	0	0
4	.120	.104	.088	.072	.056	.040	.024	.008	0	0	0
5	.150	.134	.118	.102	.086	.070	.054	.038	.022	.006	0
6	.180	.164	.148	.132	.116	.100	.084	.068	.052	.036	.020
7	.210	.194	.178	.162	.146	.130	.114	.098	.082	.066	.050
8	.240	.224	.208	.192	.176	.160	.144	.128	.112	.096	.080
9	.270	.254	.238	.222	.206	.190	.174	.158	.142	.126	.110
10	.300	.284	.268	.252	.236	.220	.204	.188	.172	.156	.140
11	.330	.314	.298	.282	.266	.250	.234	.218	.202	.186	.170
12	.360	.344	.328	.312	.296	.280	.264	.248	.232	.216	.200
13	.390	.374	.358	.342	.326	.310	.294	.278	.262	.246	.230
14	.420	.404	.388	.372	.356	.340	.324	.308	.292	.276	.260
15	.450	.434	.418	.402	.386	.370	.354	.338	.322	.306	.290

BACs for 160-pound female

No. of drinks	0	1	2	3	4	5	6	7	8	9	10
						Hours					
1	.028	.012	0	0	0	0	0	0	0	0	0
2	.056	.040	.024	.008	0	0	0	0	0	0	0
3	.084	.068	.052	.036	.020	.004	0	0	0	0	0
4	.112	.096	.080	.064	.048	.032	.016	0	0	0	0
5	.141	.125	.109	.093	.077	.061	.045	.029	.013	0	0
6	.169	.153	.137	.121	.105	.089	.073	.057	.041	.025	.009
7	.197	.181	.165	.149	.133	.117	.101	.085	.069	.053	.037
8	.225	.209	.193	.177	.161	.145	.129	.113	.097	.081	.065
9	.253	.237	.221	.205	.189	.173	.157	.141	.125	.109	.093
10	.281	.265	.249	.233	.217	.201	.185	.169	.153	.137	.121
11	.309	.293	.277	.261	.245	.229	.213	.197	.181	.165	.149
12	.337	.321	.305	.289	.273	.257	.241	.225	.209	.193	.177
13	.366	.350	.334	.318	.302	.286	.270	.254	.238	.222	.206
14	.394	.378	.362	.346	.330	.314	.298	.282	.266	.250	.234
15	.422	.406	.390	.374	.358	.342	.326	.310	.294	.278	.262

BACs for 170-pound female

No. of drinks	0	1	2	3	4	5	6	7	8	9	10
						Hours					
1	.026	.010	0	0	0	0	0	0	0	0	0
2	.053	.037	.021	.005	0	0	0	0	0	0	0
3	.079	.063	.047	.031	.015	0	0	0	0	0	0
4	.106	.090	.074	.058	.042	.026	.010	0	0	0	0
5	.132	.116	.100	.084	.068	.052	.036	.020	.004	0	0
6	.159	.143	.127	.111	.095	.079	.063	.047	.031	.015	0
7	.185	.169	.153	.137	.121	.105	.089	.073	.057	.041	.025
8	.212	.196	.180	.164	.148	.132	.116	.100	.084	.068	.052
9	.238	.222	.206	.190	.174	.158	.142	.126	.110	.094	.078
10	.265	.249	.233	.217	.201	.185	.169	.153	.137	.121	.105
11	.291	.275	.259	.243	.227	.211	.195	.179	.163	.147	.131
12	.318	.302	.286	.270	.254	.238	.222	.206	.190	.174	.158
13	.344	.328	.312	.296	.280	.264	.248	.232	.216	.200	.184
14	.371	.355	.339	.323	.307	.291	.275	.259	.243	.227	.211
15	.397	.381	.365	.349	.333	.317	.301	.285	.269	.253	.237

BAC Cards for Females *(page 3 of 4)*

BACs for 180-pound female

No. of drinks	0	1	2	3	4	5	6	7	8	9	10
						Hours					
1	.025	.009	0	0	0	0	0	0	0	0	0
2	.050	.034	.018	.002	0	0	0	0	0	0	0
3	.075	.059	.043	.027	.011	0	0	0	0	0	0
4	.100	.084	.068	.052	.036	.020	.004	0	0	0	0
5	.125	.109	.093	.077	.061	.045	.029	.013	0	0	0
6	.150	.134	.118	.102	.086	.070	.054	.038	.022	.006	0
7	.175	.159	.143	.127	.111	.095	.079	.063	.047	.031	.015
8	.200	.184	.168	.152	.136	.120	.104	.088	.072	.056	.040
9	.225	.209	.193	.177	.161	.145	.129	.113	.097	.081	.065
10	.250	.234	.218	.202	.186	.170	.154	.138	.122	.106	.090
11	.275	.259	.243	.227	.211	.195	.179	.163	.147	.131	.115
12	.300	.284	.268	.252	.236	.220	.204	.188	.172	.156	.140
13	.325	.309	.293	.277	.261	.245	.229	.213	.197	.181	.165
14	.350	.334	.318	.302	.286	.270	.254	.238	.222	.206	.190
15	.375	.359	.343	.327	.311	.295	.279	.263	.247	.231	.215

BACs for 190-pound female

No. of drinks	0	1	2	3	4	5	6	7	8	9	10
						Hours					
1	.024	.008	0	0	0	0	0	0	0	0	0
2	.047	.031	.015	0	0	0	0	0	0	0	0
3	.071	.055	.039	.023	.007	0	0	0	0	0	0
4	.095	.079	.063	.047	.031	.015	0	0	0	0	0
5	.118	.102	.086	.070	.054	.038	.022	.006	0	0	0
6	.142	.126	.110	.094	.078	.062	.046	.030	.014	0	0
7	.166	.150	.134	.118	.102	.086	.070	.054	.038	.022	.006
8	.189	.173	.157	.141	.125	.109	.093	.077	.061	.045	.029
9	.213	.197	.181	.165	.149	.133	.117	.101	.085	.069	.053
10	.237	.221	.205	.189	.173	.157	.141	.125	.109	.093	.077
11	.261	.245	.229	.213	.197	.181	.165	.149	.133	.117	.101
12	.284	.268	.252	.236	.220	.204	.188	.172	.156	.140	.124
13	.308	.292	.276	.260	.244	.228	.212	.196	.180	.164	.148
14	.332	.316	.300	.284	.268	.252	.236	.220	.204	.188	.172
15	.355	.339	.323	.307	.291	.275	.259	.243	.227	.211	.195

BACs for 200-pound female

No. of drinks	0	1	2	3	4	5	6	7	8	9	10
						Hours					
1	.022	.006	0	0	0	0	0	0	0	0	0
2	.045	.029	.013	0	0	0	0	0	0	0	0
3	.068	.052	.036	.020	.004	0	0	0	0	0	0
4	.090	.074	.058	.042	.026	.010	0	0	0	0	0
5	.113	.097	.081	.065	.049	.033	.017	.001	0	0	0
6	.135	.119	.103	.087	.071	.055	.039	.023	.007	0	0
7	.158	.142	.126	.110	.094	.078	.062	.046	.030	.014	0
8	.180	.164	.148	.132	.116	.100	.084	.068	.052	.036	.020
9	.203	.187	.171	.155	.139	.123	.107	.091	.075	.059	.043
10	.225	.209	.193	.177	.161	.145	.129	.113	.097	.081	.065
11	.248	.232	.216	.200	.184	.168	.152	.136	.120	.104	.088
12	.270	.254	.238	.222	.206	.190	.174	.158	.142	.126	.110
13	.293	.277	.261	.245	.229	.213	.197	.181	.165	.149	.133
14	.315	.299	.283	.267	.251	.235	.219	.203	.187	.171	.155
15	.338	.322	.306	.290	.274	.258	.242	.226	.210	.194	.178

BACs for 210-pound female

No. of drinks	0	1	2	3	4	5	6	7	8	9	10
						Hours					
1	.021	.005	0	0	0	0	0	0	0	0	0
2	.043	.027	.011	0	0	0	0	0	0	0	0
3	.064	.048	.032	.016	0	0	0	0	0	0	0
4	.086	.070	.054	.038	.022	.006	0	0	0	0	0
5	.107	.091	.075	.059	.043	.027	.011	0	0	0	0
6	.129	.113	.097	.081	.065	.049	.033	.017	.001	0	0
7	.150	.134	.118	.102	.086	.070	.054	.038	.022	.006	0
8	.171	.155	.139	.123	.107	.091	.075	.059	.043	.027	.011
9	.193	.177	.161	.145	.129	.113	.097	.081	.065	.049	.033
10	.214	.198	.182	.166	.150	.134	.118	.102	.086	.070	.054
11	.236	.220	.204	.188	.172	.156	.140	.124	.108	.092	.076
12	.257	.241	.225	.209	.193	.177	.161	.145	.129	.113	.097
13	.279	.263	.247	.231	.215	.199	.183	.167	.151	.135	.119
14	.300	.284	.268	.252	.236	.220	.204	.188	.172	.156	.140
15	.321	.305	.289	.273	.257	.241	.225	.209	.193	.177	.161

BAC Cards for Females (page 4 of 4)

BACs for 220-pound female

No. of drinks	Hours 0	1	2	3	4	5	6	7	8	9	10
1	.020	.004	0	0	0	0	0	0	0	0	0
2	.041	.025	.009	0	0	0	0	0	0	0	0
3	.061	.045	.029	.013	0	0	0	0	0	0	0
4	.082	.066	.050	.034	.018	.002	0	0	0	0	0
5	.102	.086	.070	.054	.038	.022	.006	0	0	0	0
6	.123	.107	.091	.075	.059	.043	.027	.011	0	0	0
7	.143	.127	.111	.095	.079	.063	.047	.031	.015	0	0
8	.164	.148	.132	.116	.100	.084	.068	.052	.036	.020	.004
9	.184	.168	.152	.136	.120	.104	.088	.072	.056	.040	.024
10	.205	.189	.173	.157	.141	.125	.109	.093	.077	.061	.045
11	.225	.209	.193	.177	.161	.145	.129	.113	.097	.081	.065
12	.245	.229	.213	.197	.181	.165	.149	.133	.117	.101	.085
13	.266	.250	.234	.218	.202	.186	.170	.154	.138	.122	.106
14	.286	.270	.254	.238	.222	.206	.190	.174	.158	.142	.126
15	.307	.291	.275	.259	.243	.227	.211	.195	.179	.163	.147

BACs for 230-pound female

No. of drinks	Hours 0	1	2	3	4	5	6	7	8	9	10
1	.020	.004	0	0	0	0	0	0	0	0	0
2	.039	.023	.007	0	0	0	0	0	0	0	0
3	.059	.043	.027	.011	0	0	0	0	0	0	0
4	.078	.062	.046	.030	.014	0	0	0	0	0	0
5	.098	.082	.066	.050	.034	.018	.002	0	0	0	0
6	.117	.101	.085	.069	.053	.037	.021	.005	0	0	0
7	.137	.121	.105	.089	.073	.057	.041	.025	.009	0	0
8	.157	.141	.125	.109	.093	.077	.061	.045	.029	.013	0
9	.176	.160	.144	.128	.112	.096	.080	.064	.048	.032	.016
10	.196	.180	.164	.148	.132	.116	.100	.084	.068	.052	.036
11	.215	.199	.183	.167	.151	.135	.119	.103	.087	.071	.055
12	.235	.219	.203	.187	.171	.155	.139	.123	.107	.091	.075
13	.254	.238	.222	.206	.190	.174	.158	.142	.126	.110	.094
14	.274	.258	.242	.226	.210	.194	.178	.162	.146	.130	.114
15	.293	.277	.261	.245	.229	.213	.197	.181	.165	.149	.133

BACs for 240-pound female

No. of drinks	Hours 0	1	2	3	4	5	6	7	8	9	10
1	.019	.003	0	0	0	0	0	0	0	0	0
2	.038	.022	.006	0	0	0	0	0	0	0	0
3	.056	.040	.024	.008	0	0	0	0	0	0	0
4	.075	.059	.043	.027	.011	0	0	0	0	0	0
5	.094	.078	.062	.046	.030	.014	0	0	0	0	0
6	.113	.097	.081	.065	.049	.033	.017	.001	0	0	0
7	.131	.115	.099	.083	.067	.051	.035	.019	.003	0	0
8	.150	.134	.118	.102	.086	.070	.054	.038	.022	.006	0
9	.169	.153	.137	.121	.105	.089	.073	.057	.041	.025	.009
10	.188	.172	.156	.140	.124	.108	.092	.076	.060	.044	.028
11	.206	.190	.174	.158	.142	.126	.110	.094	.078	.062	.046
12	.225	.209	.193	.177	.161	.145	.129	.113	.097	.081	.065
13	.244	.228	.212	.196	.180	.164	.148	.132	.116	.100	.084
14	.263	.247	.231	.215	.199	.183	.167	.151	.135	.119	.103
15	.281	.265	.249	.233	.217	.201	.185	.169	.153	.137	.121

BACs for 250-pound female

No. of drinks	Hours 0	1	2	3	4	5	6	7	8	9	10
1	.018	.002	0	0	0	0	0	0	0	0	0
2	.036	.020	.004	0	0	0	0	0	0	0	0
3	.054	.038	.022	.006	0	0	0	0	0	0	0
4	.072	.056	.040	.024	.008	0	0	0	0	0	0
5	.090	.074	.058	.042	.026	.010	0	0	0	0	0
6	.108	.092	.076	.060	.044	.028	.012	0	0	0	0
7	.126	.110	.094	.078	.062	.046	.030	.014	0	0	0
8	.144	.128	.112	.096	.080	.064	.048	.032	.016	0	0
9	.162	.146	.130	.114	.098	.082	.066	.050	.034	.018	.002
10	.180	.164	.148	.132	.116	.100	.084	.068	.052	.036	.020
11	.198	.182	.166	.150	.134	.118	.102	.086	.070	.054	.038
12	.216	.200	.184	.168	.152	.136	.120	.104	.088	.072	.056
13	.234	.218	.202	.186	.170	.154	.138	.122	.106	.090	.074
14	.252	.236	.220	.204	.188	.172	.156	.140	.124	.108	.092
15	.270	.254	.238	.222	.206	.190	.174	.158	.142	.126	.110

APPENDIX K

Alcohol Pop Quiz

BRIEF DESCRIPTION

The Alcohol Pop Quiz is a 10-item true/false quiz about the effects and dangers of alcohol.

TYPICAL APPLICATION

The Alcohol Pop Quiz is used to structure a group discussion about alcohol, including pharmacology, tolerance, blood alcohol levels, risk factors, and consumption levels. See Chapters 6 (p. 76) and 7 (p. 116).

ADMINISTRATIVE ISSUES

Time to administer: 5–20 minutes, with discussion
Time to score/interpret: n/a

COPYRIGHT ISSUES

Permission to copy? ☒ yes   ☐ no

REFERENCES

See collegedrinkingprevention.gov/facts
See www.factsontap.org
See www.jointogether.com

Alcohol Pop Quiz

Please answer "true" or "false."

_____ 1. Alcohol is classified as a "depressant" drug.

_____ 2. Individual tolerance to alcohol is one factor in calculating blood alcohol concentration (BAC).

_____ 3. Vigorous activity, cold showers, and caffeine are effective ways to get alcohol out of the bloodstream.

_____ 4. The liver can process alcohol at a rate of about two to three drinks per hour.

_____ 5. A man and woman who have the same weight and drinking history will reach the same BAC given a measured amount of alcohol.

_____ 6. In a variety of replicated studies, family history has proven to be a risk factor for developing problems with alcohol.

_____ 7. Drinking on a full stomach will prevent me from getting wasted.

_____ 8. It's impossible to overdose on alcohol.

_____ 9. There is no nutritional value to alcohol.

_____ 10. Most college students drink alcohol.

Alcohol Pop Quiz Answers and Explanation

__T__ 1. Alcohol is classified as a "depressant" drug.

Alcohol is a central nervous system depressant. However, with low doses of alcohol, and with rising blood alcohol levels, most people experience alcohol as *stimulating*. This means that at relatively low BAC levels (about .04–.06), and when first beginning to drink, most people feel more active or "buzzed." Beyond this relatively low dose, however, alcohol's *depressant* effects begin to take over. Decision making and judgment begin to be impaired, along with motor skills and reaction time. At higher doses, alcohol starts affecting other regions of the brain that control basic physiological functions such as heart rate, respiration, and blood pressure.

__F__ 2. Individual tolerance to alcohol is one factor in calculating blood alcohol concentration (BAC).

Tolerance does not affect estimation of BAC. Tolerance refers to how people feel *at a given BAC*. Alcohol is metabolized by the liver at a relatively constant rate. Individuals do vary somewhat in their ability to process alcohol, but once alcohol is in the bloodstream, there is nothing that can be done to speed up the process of elimination. By and large, BAC is a function of the amount of alcohol consumed and the time over which it was consumed. Other factors, such as weight, sex, whether alcohol is taken with food or in combination with birth control pills or other medications, or whether the alcohol contains carbon dioxide (e.g., bubbles, like those in champagne, speed up the absorption process) can also affect BAC. However, higher tolerance actually means that a person feels less at a given BAC. This means that a person needs *more* alcohol *to feel the same effects* as others. A high tolerance increases the risk of internal organ damage, risky choices (e.g., drinking and driving), and long-term health problems.

__F__ 3. Vigorous activity, cold showers, and caffeine are effective ways to get alcohol out of the bloodstream.

Once alcohol is in the bloodstream, there is nothing a person can do to speed up the process of elimination. Some factors, such as coffee or other stimulants, exercise, or a cold shower, often believed to help a person to sober up, have no effect on BAC at all. What they do is give the person a false impression of *feeling* more awake and alert—hence, the term "wide awake drunk."

__F__ 4. The liver can process alcohol at a rate of about two to three drinks per hour.

The liver breaks down alcohol at the rate of about one standard drink per hour. A standard drink, about half an ounce of ethyl alcohol, is approximately the amount of alcohol in a 12-ounce beer, 4-ounce glass of wine, or one shot of liquor. All three of these drinks contain approximately the same amount of alcohol. Of course, some "drinks" may contain much more than half an ounce of alcohol, e.g., micro-brewed or imported beers, fortified wine, or harder alcohol (e.g., Everclear, many mixed drinks, "trashcan" punch). For instance, if a man drank Thursday night and went to sleep at 2:00 A.M. with a BAC of .20, he would still be legally intoxicated (BAC of .09) at 9:30 the next morning. His BAC would not return to .00 until nearly 4 P.M. that afternoon.

(continued)

__F__ 5. A man and woman who have the same weight and drinking history will reach the same BAC given a measured amount of alcohol.

Men and women process alcohol differently. The most important difference seems to be the level of water in men's and women's bodies. Alcohol is water soluble (as opposed to other drugs like marijuana that are *fat* soluble), which means it is absorbed into parts of the body that contain water. Men have a higher proportion of body water, compared to women. Given that most men weigh more than most women (on average), men have much more body water with which to dilute alcohol. A 140-pound women who tries to keep up with a 180-pound man will likely reach *twice* as high a BAC. Other factors also conspire against women. Men have higher levels of a stomach enzyme that starts to break down alcohol before women's bodies break it down. Birth control pills and menstrual cycle may also affect how quickly alcohol is broken down. In particular, 1 week prior to menstruating, women seem to maintain peak BAC levels longer than at other times of the month.

__T__ 6. In a variety of replicated studies, family history has proven to be a risk factor for developing problems with alcohol.

People who have blood relatives with a history of alcohol or drug problems are at higher risk themselves. The risk goes up more if the relatives are more numerous, the same gender, and/or more closely related. This is particularly true among men. Researchers are not completely sure why this is the case, but it does appear that there is a strong genetic component that is inherited. In particular, a person's level of response to alcohol (i.e., high tolerance), which is partially inherited, seems to be linked to alcohol problems in later life. Those with a high family risk score *and* a high tolerance are at the greatest risk of all.

__F__ 7. Drinking on a full stomach will prevent me from getting wasted.

When alcohol is mixed with food, it takes longer for the body to absorb the alcohol. In this sense, food is acting as a buffer, slowing absorption. However, the presence of food will definitely not prevent anyone from getting wasted. All the alcohol in the stomach will eventually be absorbed into the bloodstream. Nevertheless, some have found that it is helpful to eat a meal before they go out for an evening. Not only will this slow the rate of absorption into the bloodstream, but a full stomach may also help a person to feel less like drinking because he or she will not be receiving "fill me" cues from an empty stomach. Other people have found that it is helpful to alternate drinking between alcoholic and nonalcoholic beverages. In addition to helping to moderate the amount of alcohol that gets into the bloodstream, drinking plenty of water keeps the body hydrated (alcohol is a diuretic, resulting in net loss of fluids).

__F__ 8. It's impossible to overdose on alcohol.

Each year, a number of college students die directly from alcohol consumption. Because alcohol is a depressant, it slows vital functions like breathing and heart rate and lowers blood pressure. A very high BAC can suppress breathing, heart rate, or vomiting to the point where they stop. It's also important to understand that a person's BAC may continue to rise after he or she has passed out. After a person stops drinking, alcohol in the stomach and intestine continues to be absorbed into the bloodstream. This may cause a fatal dose in someone after he or she has passed out. Other students who have been left alone after passing out have aspirated—choked—on their own vomit.

(continued)

So, it's important to stay with someone who might have had too much to drink and not to assume that he or she will be fine after sleeping it off. If you suspect that someone might be at risk for alcohol poisoning, or he or she is showing signs of confusion, vomiting, seizures, slow or irregular breathing, blue/pale skin, or he or she cannot be awakened, you should immediately call 911 for help.

___T___ 9. There is no nutritional value to alcohol.

Well, sort of. Alcoholic drinks do have calories, and, thus, provide the body with energy. A typical light beer contains about 100 calories, with sweeter drinks typically containing more. This means that it takes about 3 light beers to equal the calories of a McDonald's cheeseburger or 7 light beers to equal the calories in a pint of Ben & Jerry's cookie dough ice cream. However, the alcohol in the drink does not provide any additional vitamins or nutrients. This is why alcohol is commonly called "empty calories," because it contains no minerals, vitamins, or other basic nutrients. The danger is that the calories in alcohol fool you into thinking that your nutritional needs are being met when they are not. Consuming large amounts of alcohol can make it difficult to maintain a good diet.

___T___ 10. Most college students drink alcohol.

Most students do drink alcohol, but most are moderate drinkers. Only a minority engage in heavy or problematic drinking. Research on colleges around the country has shown that there is a tendency for students, and even faculty and staff, to overestimate the number of students who drink heavily and use other drugs. In general, men drink more than women. Groups that tend to drink more than average include students affiliated with Greek organizations, athletes, gay and lesbian students, and freshmen. Current research indicates that, on average, college men who drink five or more standard drinks in a day and college women who drink four or more per day are at a higher risk for health, academic, and social problems.

APPENDIX L

Problem-Solving Scenarios

BRIEF DESCRIPTION

The Problem-Solving Scenarios are five drinking-related scenarios that are common to the college experience.

TYPICAL APPLICATION

The Problem-Solving Scenarios are used to give students practice in problem solving and structure a group discussion about ways to intervene in high-risk situations. See Chapter 7 (p. 119).

ADMINISTRATIVE ISSUES

Time to administer: 10–20 minutes, with discussion
Time to score/interpret: n/a

COPYRIGHT ISSUES

Permission to copy?　☒ yes　☐ no

REFERENCES

n/a

Problem-Solving Scenarios

You are at a bar with a group of friends. It is near the end of a night when you have all been drinking. You see a female friend about to leave with a man you don't know. What do you do?

You are at a party and see a friend passed out on the couch. This is the first time you've seen him tonight, so you're unsure how much he's had to drink. What do you do?

One of your roommates has been acting strange lately (stranger than normal), and you think it may have something to do with alcohol. He has been partying a lot and drinking more than usual at parties. While he used to drink only on the weekends, you've noticed that he seems to be getting drunk most nights. You've also noticed that he has been skipping the morning class that both of you are enrolled in. What do you do?

You stop by a party to pick something up from a friend. You are there for about 5 minutes when you see an acquaintance with keys, obviously intoxicated, heading to his car. There are two others with him who also look like they've been drinking. What do you do? What if you were the host of the party? How (if at all) would this change your response?

Your younger brother, Paul, is a junior in high school. You know that he drinks on the weekends and occasionally smokes pot, but as far as you know Paul has never had a problem with either of these substances. One night, your parents tell you that Paul has been getting into trouble at school, skipping classes, sneaking out at night, and has come home drunk several times. They also found a stash of pot in Paul's room, but they haven't confronted him about this yet. They ask your advice about how to approach Paul. What do you tell them?

APPENDIX M

Strategies for Low-Risk Drinking

BRIEF DESCRIPTION

Presented are several strategies for moderating drinking. Students are asked to identify which might work for them.

TYPICAL APPLICATION

To help students to identify strategies and/or to initiate a conversation about changes in drinking. See Chapters 6 (p. 81) and 7 (p. 120).

ADMINISTRATIVE ISSUES

Time to administer: 5–10 minutes
Time to score/interpret: n/a

COPYRIGHT ISSUES

Permission to copy?   ☒ yes   ☐ no

REFERENCES

n/a

Strategies for Low-Risk Drinking

Students often find that it is helpful to have a plan for reducing their drinking-related risk. Which of the following strategies are likely to work for you?

- Count the number of standard drinks consumed each hour (*raises awareness of drinking*)
- Consume alcohol more slowly and/or space drinks over time (*helps pace drinking*)
- Alternate between alcoholic and nonalcoholic beverages (*helps pace drinking*)
- Set a BAC limit of no more than .05 (*keeps drinking at a moderate level*)
- Eat something before starting to drink (*helps moderate the amount of alcohol that gets into the bloodstream*)
- Avoid drinking games and doing shots (*helps keep drinking at a moderate level*)
- Spend more time with friends who don't drink (*creates more opportunities for sober events*)
- Ask a friend to accompany you and hold you accountable to responsible drinking (*serves as a reminder of commitments and a safety net*)
- Tell a few friends about the commitment not to drink heavily and ask them to help you stick to your goal (*helps solidify commitments and encourages others*)
- Engage in more activities that don't involve alcohol (*gives more alternatives to drinking*)
- Enroll in Friday classes (*keeps weekend partying from starting on Thursday night*)
- Count the number of standard drinks consumed each hour (*raises awareness of drinking*)

My choice for the next week/month (circle one) is:

Strategy	Plan
1.	
2.	
3.	

APPENDIX N

Goal Setting

BRIEF DESCRIPTION

Students are helped to identify specific changes they would like to make, as well as the reasons for those changes.

TYPICAL APPLICATION

To help students to identify drinking goals and/or to initiate a conversation about changes in drinking. See Chapters 6 (p. 81) and 7 (p. 120).

ADMINISTRATIVE ISSUES

Time to administer: 5–10 minutes
Time to score/interpret: n/a

COPYRIGHT ISSUES

Permission to copy? ☒ yes ☐ no

REFERENCES

n/a

Goal Setting

The specific changes I want to make are:	The most important reasons I want to make these changes are:
1.	1.
2.	2.
3.	3.

These are the actions I plan to take in the next week to accomplish my goals.

	Goal for this day	A difficult situation might be . . .	What I plan to do	People who will help me
Monday				
Tuesday				
Wednesday				
Thursday				
Friday				
Saturday				
Sunday				

References

Addiction Technology Transfer Center. (2004). *The change book: A blueprint for technology transfer* (2nd ed.). Kansas City, MO: Author.

Aertgeerts, B., Buntinx, F., Bande-Knops, J., Vandermeulen, C., Roelants, M., Ansoms, S., & Fevery, J. (2000). Value of CAGE, CUGE, and AUDIT in screening for alcohol abuse and dependence among college freshmen. *Alcoholism: Clinical and Experimental Research, 24*(1), 53–57.

Agostinelli, G., Brown, J. M., & Miller, W. R. (1995). Effects of normative feedback on consumption among heavy drinking college students. *Journal of Drug Education, 25*(1), 31–40.

Allison, J. (2001). *Health behaviour change: A selection of strategies* [Videotape]. Cardiff, UK: Media Resources Centre, University of Wales College of Medicine.

American Psychiatric Association. (1994). *Diagnostic and statistical manual of mental disorders* (4th ed.). Washington, DC: Author.

Amrhein, P. C., Miller, W. R., Yahne, C. E., Palmer, M., & Fulcher L. (2003). Client commitment language during motivational interviewing predicts drug use outcomes. *Journal of Consulting and Clinical Psychology, 71*(5), 862–878.

Anthony, J. C., & Arria, A. M. (1999). Epidemiology of substance abuse in adulthood. In P. J. Ott, R. E. Tarter, & R. T. Ammerman (Eds.), *Sourcebook on substance abuse: Etiology, epidemiology, assessment, and treatment* (pp. 32–49). New York: Allyn & Bacon.

Arnett, J. J. (2000). Emerging adulthood: A theory of development from the late teens through the twenties. *American Psychologist, 55*(5), 469–480.

Babor, T. F., Brown, J., & Del Boca, F. K. (1990). Validity of self-reports in applied research on addictive behaviors: Fact or fiction? *Behavioral Assessment, 12*(1), 5–31.

Baer, J. S. (2002). Student factors: Understanding individual variation in college drinking. *Journal of Studies on Alcohol* (Suppl. 14), 40–53.

Baer, J. S., & Carney, M. M. (1993). Biases in the perceptions of the consequences of alcohol use among college students. *Journal of Studies on Alcohol, 54*(1), 54–60.

Baer, J. S., Kivlahan, D. R., Blume, A. W., McKnight, P., & Marlatt, G. A. (2001). Brief intervention for heavy drinking college students: Four-year follow-up and natural history. *American Journal of Public Health, 91*(8), 1310–1316.

Baer, J. S., MacLean, M. G., & Marlatt, G. A. (1998). Linking etiology and treatment for adolescent substance abuse: Toward a better match. In R. Jessor (Ed.), *New Perspectives on Adolescent Risk Behavior* (pp. 182–220). Cambridge, UK: Cambridge University Press.

Baer, J. S., Marlatt, G. A., Kivlahan, D. R., Fromme, K., Larimer, M., & Williams, E. (1992). An experimental test of three methods of alcohol risk reduction with young adults. *Journal of Consulting and Clinical Psychology, 60*(6), 974–979.

Baer, J. S., Rosengren, D. B., Dunn, C. W., Wells, E. A, Ogle, R. L., & Hartzler, B. (2004). An evaluation of workshop training in motivational interviewing for addiction and mental health clinicians. *Drug and Alcohol Dependence, 73*(1), 99–106.

Baer, J. S., Stacy, A., & Larimer, M. (1991). Biases in the perception of drinking norms among college students. *Journal of Studies on Alcohol, 52*(6), 580–586.

Banyard, P. (2002). *Psychology in practice.* Abingon, UK: Hodder & Stoughton.

Barnett, N. P., Tevyaw, T. O., Fromme, K., Borsari, B., Carey. K. B., Corbin, W. R., Colby, S. M, & Monti, P. M. (2004). Brief alcohol interventions with mandated or adjudicated college students. *Alcoholism: Clinical and Experimental Research, 28*(6), 966–975.

Borsari, B., & Carey, K. B. (2000). Effects of a brief motivational intervention with college student drinkers. *Journal of Consulting and Clinical Psychology, 68*(4), 728–733.

Bradley, K. A., Bush, K. R., Epler, A. J., Dobie, D. J., Davis, T. M., Sporleder, J. L., Maynard, C., Burman, M. L., & Kivlahan, D. R. (2003). Two brief alcohol-screening tests from the Alcohol Use Disorders Identification Test (AUDIT). *Archives of Internal Medicine, 163*(7), 821–829.

Burke, B. L., Arkowitz, H., & Dunn, C. (2002). The efficacy of Motivational Interviewing and its adaptations: What we know so far. In W. R. Miller & S. Rollnick, *Motivational interviewing: Preparing people for change* (2nd ed., pp. 217–250). New York: Guilford Press.

Cahalan, D., Cisin, I. H., & Crossley, H. M. (1969). *American drinking practices: A national study of drinking behavior and attitudes* (Monographs of the Rutgers Center of Alcohol Studies, No. 6). New Brunswick, NJ: Rutgers Center for Alcohol Studies.

Carey, K. B., & Correia, C. J. (1997). Drinking motives predict alcohol problems in college students. *Journal of Studies on Alcohol, 58*, 100–105.

Carey, K. B., Purnine, D. M., Maisto, S. A., & Carey, M. P. (1999). Assessing readiness to change substance abuse: A critical review of instruments. *Clinical Psychology: Science and Practice, 6*(3), 245–266.

Cashin, J. R., Presley, C. A., & Meilman, P. W. (1998). Alcohol use in the Greek system: Follow the leader? *Journal of Studies on Alcohol, 59*(1), 63–70.

Chan, A. W. K., Pristach, E. A., Welte, J. W., & Russell, M. (1993). Use of the TWEAK test screening for alcoholism/heavy drinking in three populations. *Alcoholism: Clinical and Experimental Research, 17*(6), 1188–1192.

Clements, R. (1998). Critical evaluation of several alcohol screening instruments using the CIDI-SAM as a criterion measure. *Alcoholism: Clinical and Experimental Research, 22*(5), 985–993.

Collins, R. L., Parks, G. A., & Marlatt, G. A. (1985). Social determinants of alcohol consumption: The effects of social interaction and model status on the self-administration of alcohol. *Journal of Consulting and Clinical Psychology, 53*(2), 189–200.

Collins, S. E., Carey, K. B., & Sliwinski, M. J. (2002). Mailed personalized normative feedback as a brief intervention for at-risk college drinkers. *Journal of Studies on Alcohol, 63*(5), 559–567.

Connors, G. J., Donovan, D. M., & DiClemente, C. C. (2001). *Substance abuse treatment and the stages of change: Selecting and planning interventions.* New York: Guilford Press.

Connors, G. J., & Volk, R. J. (2004). Self-report screening for alcohol problems among adults. In National Institute on Alcohol Abuse and Alcoholism, *Assessing alcohol problems: A guide for clinicians and researchers* (pp. 21–36). Bethesda, MD: Author.

Curry, S. J., & Kim, E. L. (1999). Public health perspective on addictive behavior change interventions: Conceptual frameworks and guiding principles. In J. A. Tucker, D. M. Donovan, & G. A. Marlatt (Eds.), *Changing addictive behavior: Bridging clinical and public health strategies* (pp. 221–250). New York: Guilford Press.

Darkes, J, & Goldman, M. S. (1993). Expectancy challenge and drinking reduction: Experimental evidence for a mediational process. *Journal of Consulting and Clinical Psychology, 61*(2), 344–353.

Dawson, D. A., & Room, R. (2000). Towards agreement on ways to measure and report drinking patterns and alcohol-related problems in adult general population surveys: Skarpo conference overview. *Journal of Substance Abuse, 12*(1–2), 1–22.

DeJong, W. (2001). Finding common ground for effective campus-based prevention. *Psychology of Addictive Behaviors, 15*(4), 292–296.

DeJong, W., & Langford, L. M. (2002). Typology for campus-based alcohol prevention: Moving toward environmental management strategies. *Journal of Studies on Alcohol* (Suppl. 14), 140–147.

Del Boca, F. K., Darkes, J., Greenbaum, P. E., & Goldman, M. S. (2004). Up close and personal: Temporal variability in the drinking of individual college students during their first year. *Journal of Consulting and Clinical Psychology, 72*, 155–164.

DiClemente, C. C., Prochaska, J. O., Fairhurst, S. K., Velicer, W. F., Velasquez, M. M., & Rossi, J. S. (1991). The process of smoking cessation: An analysis of precontemplation, contemplation, and preparation stages of change. *Journal of Consulting and Clinical Psychology, 59*(2), 295–304.

Dimeff, L. A., Baer, J. S., Kivlahan, D. R., & Marlatt, G. A. (1999). *Brief alcohol screening and intervention for college students: A harm reduction approach.* New York: Guilford Press.

Diwan, S., & Littrell, J. (1996). Impact of small group dynamics on focus group data: Implications for social work research. *Journal of Applied Social Sciences, 20*(2), 95–106.

Donovan, D. M. (2004). Assessment to aid in the treatment planning process. In National Institute on Alcohol Abuse and Alcoholism, *Assessing alcohol problems: A guide for clinicians and researchers* (pp. 125–188). Bethesda, MD: Author.

Dunn, C. (2003). Brief motivational interviewing interventions targeting substance abuse in the acute care medical setting. *Semin Clin Neuropsychiatry, 8*(3), 188–196.

Emmen, M. J., Schippers, G. M., Bleijenberg, G., & Wollersheim, H. (2004). Effectiveness of opportunistic brief interventions for problem drinking in a general hospital setting: Systematic review. *British Medical Journal, 328*(7435), 318.

Engs, R. C., Diebold, B. A., & Hansen, D. J. (1996). The drinking patterns and problems of a national sample of college students, 1994. *Journal of Alcohol and Drug Education 41*, 13–33.

Ewing, J. A. (1984). Detecting alcoholism: The CAGE questionnaire. *Journal of the American Medical Association, 252*(14), 1905–1907.

Finney, J. W., Moos, R. H., & Timko, C. (1999). The course of treated and untreated substance use disorders: Remission and resolution, relapse and mortality. In B. S. McCrady & E. E. Epstein (Eds.), *Addictions: A comprehensive guidebook* (pp. 30–49). New York: Oxford University Press.

First, M. B., Spitzer, R. L., Gibbon, M., & Williams, J. B. W. (1995). *Structured clinical interview for DSM-IV Axis I disorders—Patient edition* (Version 2.0). New York: Biometrics Research Department, New York State Psychiatric Institute.

Flemming, M. (2002). *Clinical protocols to reduce high risk drinking in college students: The college drinking prevention curriculum for health care providers.* Bethesda, MD: National Institute on Alcohol Abuse and Alcoholism.

Forman, R. F., Svikis, D., Montoya, I. D., & Blaine, J. (2004). Selection of a substance use disorder diagnostic instrument by the National Drug Abuse Treatment Clinical Trials Network. *Journal of Substance Abuse Treatment, 27*(1),1–8.

Fromme, K., & Corbin, W. (2003). *An effective program for mandated college students.* Paper presented at the annual meeting of the Research Society on Alcoholism, Ft. Lauderdale, FL.

Fromme, K., & Corbin, W. (2004). Prevention of heavy drinking and associated negative consequences among mandated and voluntary college students. *Journal of Consulting and Clinical Psychology, 72*, 1038–1049.

Fromme, K., Stroot, E., & Kaplan, D. (1993). Comprehensive effects of alcohol: Development and psychometric assessment of a new expectancy questionnaire. *Psychological Assessment, 5*(1), 19–26.

Garvin, R. B., Alcorn, J. D., & Faulkner, K. F. (1990). Behavioral strategies for alcohol abuse prevention with high-risk college males. *Journal of Alcohol and Drug Education, 36*(1), 23–34.

Gfroerer, J. C., Greenblatt, J. C., & Wright, D. A. (1997). Substance use in the U.S. college-age population: Differences according to educational status and living arrangement. *American Journal of Public Health, 87*, 62–65.

Goldman, M. S., Greenbaum, P. E., & Darkes, J. (1997). A confirmatory test of hierarchical expectancy structure and predictive power: Discriminant validation of the alcohol expectancy questionnaire. *Psychological Assessment, 9*(2), 145–157.

Gunzerath, L., Faden, V., Zakhari, S., & Warren, K. (2004). National Institute on Alcohol Abuse and Alcoholism report on moderate drinking. *Alcoholism: Clinical and Experimental Research, 28*(6), 829–847.

Ham, L. S., & Hope, D. A. (2003). College students and problematic drinking: A review of the literature. *Clinical Psychology Review, 23*(5), 719–759.

Heck, E. J., & Lichtenberg, J. W. (1990). Validity of the CAGE in screening for problem drinking in college students. *Journal of College Student Development, 31*(4), 359–364.

Hettema, J., Steele, J., & Miller, W. R. (2005). Motivational Interviewing. *Annual Reviews in Clinical Psychology, 1,* 4.1–4.21.

Hingson, R. W., Heeren, T., Zakocs, R. C., Kopstein, A., & Wechsler, H. (2002). Magnitude of alcohol-related mortality and morbidity among U.S. college students ages 18–24. *Journal of Studies on Alcohol, 63*(2), 136–144.

Hingson, R. W., & Howland, J. (2002). Comprehensive community interventions to promote health: Implications for college-age drinking problems. *Journal of Studies on Alcohol* (Suppl. 14), 226–240.

Hudziak, J. J., Helzer, J. E, Wetzel, M. W., Kessel, K. B., McGee, B., Janca, A., & Przybeck, T. (1993). The use of the DSM-III-R Checklist for initial diagnostic assessments. *Comprehensive Psychiatry, 34*(6), 375–383.

Hurlbut, S. C., & Sher, K. J. (1992). Assessing alcohol problems in college students. *Journal of American College Health, 41* (2), 49–58.

Ingersoll, K. S., Wagner, C. C., & Gharib, S. (2000). *Motivational groups for community substance abuse programs.* Richmond, VA: Mid-Atlantic Addictions Technology Transfer Center.

Jessor, R., Donovan, J. E., & Costa, F. M. (1991). *Beyond adolescence: Problem behavior and young adult development.* Cambridge, UK: Cambridge University Press.

Johnston, L. D., O'Malley, P. M., & Bachman, J. G. (2001). *Monitoring the Future. National survey results on drug use, 1975–2000: Vol. II. College students and adults ages 19–40.* Bethesda, MD: National Institute on Drug Abuse.

Johnston, L. D., O'Malley, P. M., & Bachman, J. G. (2002). *Monitoring the Future. National survey results on drug use, 1975–2001: Vol. II. College students and adults ages 19–40.* Bethesda, MD: National Institute on Drug Abuse.

Kahler, C. W., Strong, D. R., Read, J. P., Palfai, T. P., & Wood, M.D. (2004). Mapping the continuum of alcohol problems in college students: A Rasch model analysis. *Psychology of Addictive Behaviors, 18*(4), 322–333.

Kitchens, J. M. (1994). Does this patient have an alcohol problem? *Journal of the American Medical Association, 272*(22), 1782–1787.

Knight, J. R., Wechsler, H., Kuo, M., Seibring, M., Weitzman, E. R., & Schuckit, M. A. (2002). Alcohol abuse and dependence among U.S. college students. *Journal of Studies on Alcohol, 63*(3), 263–270.

Kokotailo, P. K., Egan, J., Gangnon, R., Brown, D., Mundt, M., & Fleming, M. (2004). Validity of the Alcohol Use Disorders Identification Test in college students. *Alcoholism: Clinical and Experimental Research, 28,* 914–920.

Kushner, M. G., Sher, K. J., & Erickson, D. J. (1999). Prospective analysis of the relation between DSM-III anxiety disorders and alcohol use disorders. *American Journal of Psychiatry, 156*(5), 723–732.

Kypri, K., & Langley, J. D. (2003). Perceived social norms and their relation to university student drinking. *Journal of Studies on Alcohol, 64,* 829–835.

Lane, C., Huws-Thomas, M., Hood, K., Rollnick, S., Edwards, K., & Robling, M. (2005). Measuring adaptations of motivational interviewing: The development and validation of the Behavior Change Counseling Index (BECCI). *Patient Education and Counseling, 56*(2), 166–173.

Larimer, M. E., & Cronce, J. M. (2002). Identification, prevention, and treatment: A review of individual-focused strategies to reduce problematic alcohol consumption by college students. *Journal of Studies on Alcohol* (Suppl 14), 148–163.

Larimer, M. E., Irvine, D. L., Kilmer, J. R., & Marlatt, G. A. (1997). College drinking and the Greek system: Examining the role of perceived norms for high-risk behavior. *Journal of College Student Development, 38*(6), 587–598.

Larimer, M. E., Lydum, A., Anderson, B., & Turner, A. (1999). Male and female recipients of unwanted sexual contact in a college student sample: Prevalence rates, alcohol use, and depressive symptoms. *Sex Roles, 40,* 295–308.

Larimer, M. E., Turner, A. P., Anderson, B. K., Fader, J. S., Kilmer, J. R., Palmer, R. S., & Cronce, J. M. (2001). Evaluating a brief alcohol intervention with fraternities. *Journal of Studies on Alcohol, 62*(3), 370–380.

Leichliter, J. S., Meilman, P. W., Presley, C. A., & Cashin, J. R. (1998). Alcohol use and related consequences among students with varying levels of involvement in college athletics. *Journal of American College Health, 46*(6), 257–262.

Look, S., & Rapaport, R. J. (1991). Evaluation of an alcohol education discipline program for college students. *Journal of Alcohol and Drug Education, 36*(2), 88–95.

Maddock, J. E., Laforge, R. G., Rossi, J. S., & O'Hare, T. (2001). The college alcohol problems scale. *Addictive Behaviors, 26*(3), 385–398.

Maisto, S. A., & Connors, G. J. (1990). Clinical diagnostic techniques and assessment tools in alcohol research. *Alcohol Health and Research World, 14*(3), 232–238.

Maisto, S. A., McKay, J. R., & Tiffany, S. T. (2004). Diagnosis. In National Institute on Alcohol Abuse and Alcoholism, *Assessing alcohol problems: A guide for clinicians and researchers* (pp. 55–74). Bethesda, MD: Author.

Mann, R. E., Sobell, L. C., Sobell, M. B., & Pavan, D. (1985). Reliability of a family tree questionnaire for assessing family history of alcohol problems. *Drug and Alcohol Dependence, 15*(1–2), 61–67.

Marlatt, G. A., Baer, J. S., Kivlahan, D. R., Dimeff, L. A., Larimer, M. E., Quigley, L. A., Somers, J. M., & Williams, E. (1998). Screening and brief intervention for high-risk college student drinkers: Results from a two-year follow-up assessment. *Journal of Consulting and Clinical Psychology, 66*(4), 604–615.

Mayfield, D., McLeod, G., & Hall, P. (1974). CAGE questionnaire: Validation of a new alcoholism screening instrument. *American Journal of Psychiatry, 131*(10), 1121–1123.

McConnaughy, E. A., DiClemente, C. C., Prochaska, J. O., & Velicer, W. F. (1989). Stages of change in psychotherapy: A follow-up report. *Psychotherapy: Theory, Research, and Practice, 26*, 494–503.

McConnaughy, E. A., Prochaska, J. O., & Velicer, W. F. (1983). Stages of change in psychotherapy: Measurement and sample profiles. *Psychotherapy: Theory, Research, and Practice, 20*, 368–375.

Medical consequences of alcohol abuse. (2000). *Alcohol Research and Health, 24*(1), 27–31.

Miller, W. R. (2000). Rediscovering fire: Small interventions, large effects. *Psychology of Addictive Behaviors, 14*(1), 6–18.

Miller, W. R., Benefield, R. G., & Tonigan, J. S. (1993). Enhancing motivation for change in problem drinking: A controlled comparison of two therapist styles. *Journal of Consulting and Clinical Psychology, 61*, 455–461.

Miller, W. R., & C'de Baca, J. (2001). *Quantum change: When epiphanies and sudden insights transform ordinary lives.* New York: Guilford Press.

Miller, W. R., & Hester, R. K. (2003). Treatment for alcohol problems: Toward an informed eclecticism. In R. K. Hester & W. R. Miller (Eds.), *Handbook of alcoholism treatment approaches: Effective alternatives* (2nd ed., pp. 1–12). Needham Heights, MA: Allyn & Bacon.

Miller, W. R., & Pechacek, T. F. (1987). New roads: Assessing and treating psychological dependence. *Journal of Substance Abuse Treatment, 4*, 73–77.

Miller, W. R., & Rollnick, S. (2002). *Motivational interviewing: Preparing people for change* (2nd ed.). New York: Guilford Press.

Miller, W. R., & Tonigan, J. S. (1996). Assessing drinkers' motivation for change: The Stages of Change Readiness and Treatment Eagerness Scale (SOCRATES). *Psychology of Addictive Behaviors, 10*(2), 81–89.

Miller, W. R., Zweben, A., DiClemente, C. C., & Rychtarik, R. G. (1995). *Motivational Enhancement Therapy Manual: Vol. 2, Project MATCH Monograph Series.* Rockville, MD: National Institute on Alcohol Abuse and Alcoholism.

Monti, P. M., Colby, S. M., Barnett, N. P., Spirito, A. Rohsenow, D. J., Myers, M., Woolard, R., & Lewander, W. (1999). Brief intervention for harm reduction with alcohol-positive older adolescents in a hospital emergency department. *Journal of Consulting and Clinical Psychology, 67*, 989–994.

Monti, P. M., Kadden, R. M., Rohsenow, D. J., Cooney, N. L., & Abrams, D. B. (2002). *Treating alcohol dependence: A coping skills training guide.* New York: Guilford Press.

Mukamal, K. J., Conigrave, K. M., Mittleman, M. A., Camargo, C. A., Jr., Stampfer, M. J., Willett, W. C., & Rimm, E. B. (2003). Roles of drinking pattern and type of alcohol consumed in coronary heart disease in men. *New England Journal of Medicine, 348*(2), 109–118.

Murphy, J. G., Duchnick, J. J., Vuchinich, R. E., Davison, J. W., Karg, R. S., Olson, A. M., et al. (2001). Relative efficacy of a brief motivational intervention for college student drinkers. *Psychology of Addictive Behaviors, 15*(4), 373–379.

Naimi, T.S., Brewer, R.D., Mokdad, A., Denny, C., Serdula, M.K., & Marks, J.S. (2003). Binge drinking among U.S. adults. *Journal of the American Medical Association, 289*(1), 70–75.

National Institute on Alcohol Abuse and Alcoholism (NIAAA). (2002). *A call to action: Changing the culture of drinking at U.S. colleges.* Bethesda, MD: Task Force of the National Advisory Council on Alcohol Abuse and Alcoholism.

National Institute on Alcohol Abuse and Alcoholism (NIAAA). (2004). *Assessing alcohol problems: A guide for clinicians and researchers.* Bethesda, MD: Author.

Neighbors, C., Larimer, M. E., & Lewis, M. A. (2004). Targeting misperceptions of descriptive drinking norms: Efficacy of a computer-delivered personalized normative feedback intervention. *Journal of Consulting and Clinical Psychology, 72*(3), 434–447.

Neighbors, C., Walker, D. D., & Larimer, M. E. (2003). Expectancies and evaluations of alcohol effects among college students: Self-determination as a moderator. *Journal of Studies on Alcohol, 64*(2), 292–300.

Nelson, T. F., & Wechsler, H. (2003). School spirits: Alcohol and collegiate sports fans. *Addictive Behaviors, 28*(1), 1–11.

Nye, E. C., Agostinelli, G., & Smith, J. E. (1999). Enhancing alcohol problem recognition: A self-regulation model for the effects of self-focusing and normative information. *Journal of Studies on Alcohol, 60*(5), 685–693.

O'Hare, T. (1997a). Measuring excessive alcohol use in college drinking contexts: The Drinking Context Scale. *Addictive Behaviors, 22*(4), 469–477.

O'Hare, T. (1997b). Measuring problem drinking in first time offenders: Development and validation of the College Alcohol Problems Scale (CAPS). *Journal of Substance Abuse Treatment, 14*(4), 383–387.

O'Malley, P. M., & Johnston, L. D. (2002). Epidemiology of alcohol and other drug use among American college students. *Journal of Studies on Alcohol* (Suppl. 14), 23–39.

Perkins, H. W. (2002). Surveying the damages: A review of research on consequences of alcohol misuse in college populations. *Journal of Studies on Alcohol* (Suppl. 14), 91–100.

Perkins, H. W., & Berkowitz, A. D. (1986). Perceiving the community norms of alcohol use among students: Some research implications for campus alcohol education programming. *International Journal of the Addictions, 21*(9/10), 961–976.

Perz, C. A., DiClemente, C. C., & Carbonari, J. P. (1996). Doing the right thing at the right time?: The interaction of stages and processes of change in successful smoking cessation. *Health Psychology, 15*(6), 462–468.

Pokorny, A. D., Miller, B. A., & Kaplan, H. B. (1972). The brief MAST: A shortened version of the Michigan Alcoholism Screening Test. *American Journal of Psychiatry, 129*, 342–345.

Posavac, E. J. (1993). College students' views of excessive drinking and the university's role. *Journal of Drug Education, 23*(3), 237–245.

Presley, C. A., Meilman, P. W., Cashin, J. R., & Lyerla, R. (1996). *Alcohol and drugs on American college campuses: Use, consequences, and perceptions of the campus environment. Volume III: 1991–1993.* Carbondale, IL: Southern Illinois University.

Presley, C. A., Meilman, P. W., & Leichliter, J. S. (2002). College factors that influence drinking. *Journal of Studies on Alcohol* (Suppl. 14), 82–90.

Prochaska, J. O., DiClemente, C. C., & Norcross, J. C. (1992). In search of how people change: Applications to addictive behaviors. *American Psychologist, 47*(9), 1102–1114.

Robins, L. N., Wing, J., Wittchen, H. U., Helzer, J. E., Babor, T. F., Burke, J., Farmer, A., Jablensky, A., Pickens, R., Regier, D. A., Sartorius, N., & Towle, L. H. (1989). The Composite International Diagnostic Interview: An epidemiologic instrument suitable for use in conjunction with different diagnostic systems and in different cultures. *Archives of General Psychiatry, 45*, 1069–1077.

Rollnick, S. (1998). Readiness, importance, and confidence: Critical conditions of change in treatment. In W. R. Miller & N. Heather (Eds.), *Treating addictive behaviors* (2nd ed., pp. 49–60). New York: Plenum Press.

Rollnick, S., Allison, J., Ballasiotes, S., Barth, T., Butler, C. C., Rose, G. S., & Rosengren, D. B. (2002). Variations on a theme: Motivational interviewing and its adaptations. In W. R. Miller & S. Rollnick, *Motivational interviewing: Preparing people for change* (2nd ed., pp. 270–283). New York: Guilford Press.

Rollnick, S., Heather, N., Gold, R., & Hall, W. (1992). Development of a short "readiness to change" questionnaire for use in brief, opportunistic interventions among excessive drinkers. *British Journal of Addiction, 87*(5), 743–754.

Rollnick, S., Mason, P., & Butler, C. (1999). *Health behavior change: A guide for practitioners*. Edinburgh, UK: Churchill Livingstone.

Ross, H. E., Gavin, D. R., & Skinner, H. A. (1990). Diagnostic validity of the MAST and the Alcohol Dependence Scale in the assessment of DSM-III alcohol disorders. *Journal of Studies on Alcohol, 51*(6), 506–513.

Sadler, O. W., & Scott, A. M. (1993). First offenders: a systematic response to underage drinking on the college campus. *Journal of Alcohol and Drug Education, 38*(2), 62–71.

Saltz, R. F., & DeJong, W. (2002). *Reducing alcohol problems on campus: A guide to planning and evaluation*. Bethesda, MD: Task Force of the National Advisory Council on Alcohol Abuse and Alcoholism.

Saunders, J. B., Aasland, O. G., Babor, T. F., De La Fuente, J. R., & Grant, M. (1993). Development of the Alcohol Use Disorders Identification Test (AUDIT): WHO collaborative project on early detection of persons with harmful alcohol consumption. *Addiction, 88*, 791–804.

Schroeder, R. C. (2001). *High-risk drinking: A research-based approach to alcohol education on campus*. Paper presented at the annual conference of the American College Health Association, Las Vegas, NV.

Schulenberg, J. E., & Maggs J. L. (2002). A developmental perspective on alcohol use and heavy drinking during adolescence and the transition to young adulthood. *Journal of Studies on Alcohol* (Suppl. 14), 54–70.

Schulenberg, J., O'Malley, P. M., Bachman, J. G., Wadsworth, K. N., & Johnston, L. D. (1996). Getting drunk and growing up: Trajectories of frequent binge drinking during the transition to young adulthood. *Journal of Studies on Alcohol, 57*(3), 289–304.

Selzer, M. L. (1971). Michigan Alcoholism Screening Test: The quest for a new diagnostic instrument. *American Journal of Psychiatry, 127*(12), 1653–1658.

Sher, K. J., Bartholow, B. D., & Nanda, S. (2001). Short- and long-term effects of fraternity and sorority membership on heavy drinking: A social norms perspective. *Psychology of Addictive Behaviors, 15*(1), 42–51.

Skinner, H. A., & Horn, J. L. (1984). *Alcohol dependence scale (ADS) user's guide*. Toronto, Canada: Addiction Research Foundation.

Slutske, W. S., Hunt-Carter, E. E., Nabors-Oberg, R. E., Sher, K. J., Bucholz, K. K., Madden, P. A., Anokhin, A., & Heath, A. C. (2004). Do college students drink more than their non–college-attending peers? Evidence from a population-based longitudinal female twin study. *Journal of Abnormal Psychology, 113*(4), 530–540.

Smith, D. S., Collins, M., Kreisberg, J. P., Volpicelli, J. R., & Alterman, A. I. (1987). Screening for problem drinking in college freshman. *Journal of American College Health, 36*, 89–94.

Sobell, L. C., Cunningham, J. A., & Sobell, M. B. (1996). Recovery for alcoholic problems with and without treatment: Prevalence in two population surveys. *American Journal of Public Health, 86*(7), 966–972.

Sobell, L. C., & Sobell, M. B. (1992). Timeline follow-back: A technique for assessing self-reported alcohol consumption. In R. Z. Litten & J. P. Allen (Eds.), *Measuring alcohol consumption: Psychosocial and biochemical methods* (pp. 41–72). Totowa, NJ: Humana Press.

Sobell, L. C., & Sobell, M. B. (2004). Alcohol consumption measures. In National Institute on Alcohol Abuse and Alcoholism, *Assessing alcohol problems: A guide for clinicians and researchers* (pp. 75–100). Bethesda, MD: Author.

Sobell, L. C., Toneatto, T., & Sobell, M. B. (1994). Behavioral assessment and treatment planning for alcohol, tobacco, and other drug problems: Current status with an emphasis on clinical applications. *Behavior Therapy, 25*(4), 533–580.

Sobell, M. B., & Sobell, L. C. (1999). Stepped care for alcohol problems: An efficient method for planning and delivering clinical services. In J. A. Tucker, D. M. Donovan, & G. A. Marlatt (Eds.), *Changing addictive behavior: Bridging clinical and public health strategies* (pp. 331–343). New York: Guilford Press.

Sobell, M. B., & Sobell, L. C. (2000). Stepped care as a heuristic approach to the treatment of alcohol problems. *Journal of Consulting and Clinical Psychology, 68*(4), 573–579.

Straus, R., & Bacon, S. D. (1953). *Drinking in college*. New Haven, CT: Yale University Press.

Stuart, M. R., & Lieberman, J. A. (2002). *The fifteen minute hour* (3rd ed.). New York: Saunders.

Thombs, D. L., & Beck, K. H. (1994). Social context of four adolescent drinking patterns. *Health Education Research, 9*(1), 13–22.

Thombs, D. L., Olds, R. S., & Snyder, B. M. (2003). Field assessment of BAC data to study late-night college drinking. *Journal of Studies on Alcohol, 64*(3), 322–330.

Thombs, D. L., Wolcott, B. J., & Farkash, L. G. E. (1997). Social context, perceived norms and drinking behavior in young people. *Journal of Substance Abuse, 9*, 257–267.

Tonigan, J. S., Miller, W. R., & Brown, J. M. (1997). Reliability of Form 90: An instrument for assessing alcohol treatment outcome. *Journal of Studies on Alcohol, 58*(4), 358–364.

Toomey, T. L., & Wagenaar, A. C. (2002). Environmental policies to reduce college drinking: Options and research findings. *Journal of Studies on Alcohol* (Suppl. 14), 193–205.

Valliant, P. M., & Scanlan, P. (1996). Personality, living arrangements, and alcohol use by first year university students. *Social Behavior and Personality, 24*(2), 151–156.

Velasquez, M. M., Maurer, G. G., Crouch, C., & DiClemente, C. C. (2001). *Group treatment for substance abuse*. New York: Guilford Press.

Walters, S. T. (2000). In praise of feedback: An effective intervention for college students who are heavy drinkers. *Journal of American College Health, 48*, 235–238.

Walters S. T. & Bennett M. E. (2000). Addressing drinking among college students: A review of the empirical literature. *Alcoholism Treatment Quarterly, 18*(1), 61–77.

Walters, S. T., Bennett, M. E., & Miller. J. E. (2000). Reducing alcohol use in college students: A controlled trial of two brief interventions. *Journal of Drug Education, 30*(3), 361–372.

Walters, S. T., Gruenewald, D. A., Miller, J. H., & Bennett, M. E. (2001). Early findings from a disciplinary program to reduce problem drinking by college students. *Journal of Substance Abuse Treatment, 20*(1), 89–91.

Walters, S. T., & Neighbors, C. (2005). Feedback interventions for college alcohol misuse: What, why and for whom? *Addictive Behaviors, 30*, 1168–1182.

Walters, S. T., Ogle, R., & Martin, J. E. (2002). Perils and possibilities of group-based MI. In W. R. Miller & S. Rollnick (Eds.), *Motivational interviewing: Preparing people for change* (2nd ed., pp. 377–390). New York: Guilford Press.

Wechsler, H., Dowdall, G. W., Maenner, G., Gledhill-Hoyt, J., & Lee, H. (1998). Changes in binge drinking and related problems among American college students between 1993 and 1997: Results of the Harvard School of Public Health College Alcohol Study. *Journal of American College Health, 47*(9), 57–68.

Wechsler, H., Lee, J. E., Kuo, M., Seibring, M., Nelson, T. F., & Lee, H. (2002). Trends in college binge drinking during a period of increased prevention efforts. *Journal of American College Health, 50*, 203–217.

Wechsler, H., Moeykens, B., Davenport, A., Castillo, S., & Hansen, J. (1995). Adverse impact of heavy episodic drinkers on other college students. *Journal of Studies on Alcohol, 56*(6), 628–634.

Wechsler, H., Molnar, B. E., Davenport, A. E., & Baer, J. S. (1999). College alcohol use: A full or empty glass? *Journal of American College Health, 47*(6), 247–252.

Weingardt, K. R., Baer, J. S., Kivlahan, D. R., Roberts, L. J., Miller, E. T., & Marlatt, G. A. (1998). Episodic heavy drinking among college students: Methodological issues and longitudinal perspectives. *Psychology of Addictive Behaviors, 12*(3), 155–167.

Weitzman, E. R., Folkman, A., Folkman, K. L., & Wechsler, H. (2003). Relationship of alcohol outlet density to heavy and frequent drinking and drinking-related problems among college students at eight universities. *Health and Place, 9*(1), 1–6.

White, H. R., & Labouvie, E. W. (1989). Towards the assessment of adolescent problem drinking. *Journal of Studies on Alcohol, 50*(1), 30–37.

Williams, J. G., & Morrice, A. (1992). Measuring drinking patterns among college students. *Psychological Reports, 70*(1), 231–238.

Wood, M. D., Vinson, D. C., & Sher, K. J. (2001). Alcohol use and misuse. In A. Baum, T. Revenson, & J. Singer (Eds.), *Handbook of health psychology* (pp. 281–318). Hillsdale, NJ: Erlbaum.

Wood, P. K., Sher, K. J., Erickson, D. J., & DeBord, K. A. (1997). Predicting academic problems in college from freshman alcohol involvement. *Journal of Studies on Alcohol, 58*(2), 200–210.

World Health Organization Brief Intervention Study Group. (1996). A randomized cross-national clinical trial of brief interventions with heavy drinkers. *American Journal of Public Health, 86*, 948–955.

Yalom, I. (1995). *The theory and practice of group psychotherapy* (4th ed.). New York: Basic Books.

Index

Academic performance, 9
Action stage of change, 18–19
Additive risk factors, 16
Advice
  in brief interventions, 63–66
  "elicit–provide–elicit" format, 64–
    65
  example of 71–72
  menu of options for, 82
  training in, 128–129
Affirmations
  in closing a session, 80
  in motivational counseling, 50–51
  positive effects of, 51
Agenda, in group interventions,
    104–105
Aggressiveness, 9
Alcohol abuse, DSM-IV criteria, 34
Alcohol consumption, assessment,
    27–32, 40
Alcohol dependence
  assessment, 33–35
  DSM-IV criteria, 34
  rates of, 9
Alcohol Dependence Scale, 35
Alcohol poisoning, 8
"Alcohol Pop Quiz," 116, 121, 190–
    194
Alcohol screening. See Screening
Alcohol Use Disorders
    Identification Test (AUDIT),
    35–36, 40, 135–137
Ambivalence about change
  and double-sided reflections, 53–
    54, 105
  in groups, 105
  motivational exercise for, 83–85

Assessing Alcohol Problems
    (NIAAA), 26
Assessment, 25–41
  alcohol dependence, 33–35
  alcohol expectancies, 38
  consequences of drinking, 32–33
  drinking context, 38
  drinking rate, 27–32
  example of, 96–97
  family history, 39
  in initial interview, 76–78
  motivation, 37
  purpose of, 25
  screening phase, 35–36
  summary of recommendations, 40
AUDIT. See Alcohol Use Disorders
    Identification Test
AUDIT-C, 36

BAC cards, 30–31, 181–189
BAC Self-Monitoring Card, 180
BAC Zone, 30, 95
BASICS manual, 76, 86
Behavior Change Counseling
    Index, 129
Behavioral consultation
  definition, 23
  sample of, 72–73
  training in, 128–129
Behavioral Risk Factor Surveillance
    System, 5–6
Beliefs, assessment, 38
"Binge" episode. See Episodic
    heavy drinking
Biological model, 14
Blood alcohol concentration (BAC),
    30–31

Brainstorming
  discrepancy-building method, 109
  of drinking pros and cons,
    groups, 114–116
"Bravado drinker," 111
Breath analysis, 3–4
Brief interventions, 60–74
  advice and suggestions in, 23,
    63–66
    example, 71–7d2
  behavioral consultation example,
    72–73
  closing the interaction, 70–71
  in groups, 102
  long intervention differences, 61
  model of, 23
  training in, 128–129
  transitioning to alcohol concerns
    in, 61–63
Brief MAST, 35

CAGE questionnaire, screening
    use, 35
Calories consumed feedback, 86
CAPSr. See College Alcohol
    Problems Scale—Revised
"Change talk"
  and ambivalence, 58
  categories of, 57
  eliciting of, 57–58
  in readiness to change stage, 80–83
Check-Up to Go (CHUG)
    assessment, 158–170
  blood alcohol concentration, 31
  drinking rate, 29
  feedback intervention, 86
  time constraints, 96

Closed-ended questions, 49
Closing a session, 78–80
Cocaine use, survey data, 8
Cognitive-behavioral skills training, 21–22
Co-leader teams, 112–113
  and brainstorming, 115–116
  double-sided presentations, 105
  recommendations, 112–113
College Alcohol Problems Scale—Revised (CAPS-r), 144–146
  consequences of drinking assessment, 32–33, 40
  feedback function of, 86–87
  time constraints, 96
College drinking
  comparison to other groups, 4–6, 9
  gender differences in, 2–3
  problems created by, 8–10
  risk factors for, 14–16
  student attitudes toward, 10–11
  surveys of, 2
  trends, 6–7
  variability in, 3–5
Composite International Diagnostic Interview, 34
Comprehensive Effects of Alcohol scale (CEOA), 150–155
  example of use of, 98
  expectancies measure, 38, 40, 88–89
  in functional analysis, 88–89
  time constraints, 96
Computer-generated feedback, 86
Confidence in change
  motivational profile, 45–46
  tailored intervention link, 47–48
Confidence Ruler, 67–70, 156–157
Confidentiality
  explanation to student, 76–77
  in groups, 105, 113
  limits of, 76
Consequence measures, 32–33, 40
Consumption assessment, 27–32, 40
Contemplation stage of change, 18–19, 37
Contextual factors, assessment, 38, 40
Controlled drinking, in goal setting, 82–83
CORE Institute studies, 2–3, 6
CUGE questionnaire, screening use, 35

Daily diary
  drinking frequency, 3
  in self-monitoring, 93–95
Daily drinking
  ages 18–40, trends, 5–6
  assessment, 28, 30–32
  yearly trends, 7
Daily Drinking Questionnaire (DDQ), 29
Defensiveness, 76. *See also* Resistance
Depression, as risk factor, 15
Developmental factors, 16–17
Developmental transitions, 17
Diaries. *See* Daily diary
Discrepancy-building methods
  advantages and disadvantages, 109
  in groups, 108–110
Disinhibition, as risk factor, 14–15
Double-sided reflections
  in groups, 105
  and pros and cons of drinking, 84
Drinking context, assessment, 38
Drinking Context Scale, 38, 40, 96
Drinking feedback. *See* Feedback
Drinking Practices Questionnaire, 32
Drinking rate, assessment, 31–32
Driving under the influence, 8
Drug use, 8
DSM checklist, 34, 40
DSM-IV, alcohol dependence criteria, 34

Educational programs, 103
"Elicit–provide–elicit" (E-P-E) format, 64–65
Empathy
  in group format, 105
  motivational interviewing principle, 44
  training selection, 130
Environmental prevention strategies, 124–125
Environmental risk factors, 15–16
Episodic heavy drinking
  ages 18–40, trends, 5–6
  assessment, 27–32
  definition, 2
  frequency, 2–3, 9
  group discussion, 107–108
  high school and college data, 4–5
  intercollege variability, 5
  risk reduction goal, 82
  student opinions/perception, 10–11

Expectancies
  assessment, 38
  challenges to, 21–22
  functional analysis exercise, 88–91
Extraversion, 15

Family history, assessment, 39–40
Family Tree Questionnaire, 39–40
Feedback
  basic steps, 87
  difficulties in group format, 103
  discrepancy-building method, groups, 109–110, 116–118
  cautions, 110, 117
  example of, 97–98
  as motivational exercise, 86–88
  in provider training, 129–130
Fighting, 9
Forced choice activity, in groups, 114, 120–121
Form 90 measure, 30
Fraternity membership, 16
Frequency of drinking
  assessment, 27–32
  definition, 1
Functional analysis
  example of, 98
  "New Roads" activity in, 88–91, 98

Gender differences, heavy drinking, 2–3
Genetic risk factors, 15
Goal setting
  benchmarks, 82
  and self-monitoring, 95
  worksheet, 99, 199–200
"Good Things, Not-So-Good Things" exercise, 83–85
  in group format, 114–116, 121
  in individual sessions, 83–85, 97
Grade point averages, 9
Group forced choice activity, 114
  example of, 120–121
  self-disclosure function of, 114
Group interventions, 101–122
  composition of group, 112
  discrepancy-building methods, 108–110
  empathic environment in, 105
  establishing an agenda, 104–105
  facilitator rules, 104–113
  feedback in, 109–110, 116–118
  cautions, 110, 117
  problem solving, 129

rationale and challenges, 102–104
reflections and summaries in, 107–108
resistance in, 105–107, 110–111
sample of, 120–121
strategies, 113–120
training, 129

Harm-reduction strategies, 119
Heavy drinking. *See* Episodic heavy drinking
"Host" risk factors, 14
Hostile group members, 110
Hypothetical change strategy, 66–67

Importance of change
assessment, 37
motivational profiles, 44–48
tailored intervention link, 47–48
Importance Ruler, 67–70, 156–157
Impulsivity, as risk factor, 14–15
Indicated prevention, 124
Informational interventions
group format, 103
ineffectiveness, 21–22, 103
Intoxicated driving, 8

Knowledge-based interventions, 21–22

Life values exercise. *See* Values cardsort exercise

Mailed feedback, 86
Maintenance stage of change, 18–19
Marijuana use, survey data, 8
Michigan Alcoholism Screening Test (MAST), 35
Models, alcohol problems, 13–14
Moderate drinking, in goal setting, 82–83
Monitoring the Future studies, 2–3, 5–7
Moral model, 14
Motivation. *See* Readiness to change
Motivational exercises, 83–85
Motivational group, 102
Motivational intervention (MI), 42–59, 75–100
closing a session, 78–80
core interview techniques, 48–59
counseling style in, 42–59
deconstruction of, 43–44

example of, 95–99
feedback in, 86–88
as "gold standard," 24, 75
initial session, 76–77
interview general principles, 43–44
life values exercise in, 91–93
motivational exercises, 83–95
training, 129
Motivational Interviewing Treatment Integrity coding system, 129
Multiplicative risk factors, 16
Myths, college campus drinking, 117

National College Health Risk Behavior Survey, 2–3
National Institute on Alcohol Abuse and Alcohol report, 20–23
Negative consequences, drinking, 32–33, 40
"New Roads" activity, 88–91, 98
Nonparticipatory group members, 111
Norms for college drinking, 117, 121

OARS skills, 48–57
Open-ended questions
in initial interview, 77
in motivational counseling, 49–50
Organizational-level interventions, 124

Paradoxical brainstorm, 115–116
Peer alcohol use, as risk factor, 15
Physical fights, 9
Physical injuries, 8
Precontemplation stage of change, 18–19, 37
Preparation stage of change, 18–19
Preventive interventions, 124–125
Problem solving
example of, 121
in groups, 119–121
Problem-Solving Scenarios, 119, 195–196
Psychoeducational group, 102
Public health perspective, 14

Quantity–frequency methods, 28–30
Quantity of drinking
assessment, 27–32
limitations, 28–29
definition, 1

Rapport, in motivational intervention, 76–77, 78
Readiness to change
assessment, 37–38
indicators of, 80
Readiness to Change Questionnaire, 147–149
description of, 37–38, 40
time constraints, 96
"Reasons for change" exercise, 83
"Reasons for Staying the Same" exercise, 83
Reflective listening, 51–55. *See also* OARS skills
and ambivalence to change, 53–54, 84–85
and "change talk," 58
in closing a session, 78–79
"continuing the paragraph" in, 52–53
double-sided form of, 53–54
in initial interview, 77
and life values exercise, 92–93
and "rolling with" resistance, 54–55
Resistance
acknowledgement of, 76–77
in groups, 105–107, 110–111
motivational interviewing approach to, 44, 76–77
reflective listening approach, 54–55, 77
Risk factors, 14–16
Risk reduction, in goal setting, 82
Role exploration, 17
Role play, in training, 129
"Rolling with" resistant comments, 54–55
Rutgers Alcohol Problem Index, 32

Sample intervention protocols
behavioral consultation, 72–73
brief intervention, 71–72
group intervention, 120–121
motivational intervention, 96–100
Scaled questions, 67–70, 73
Screening
measures, 35–36, 40
recommendations, 36
and service integration, 126–127
Selective prevention, 124
Self-disclosure, and forced choice activity, 114
Self-efficacy, 44

Self-exploration, 17
Self-monitoring cards, 93–95, 97,
    179–180
Self-report assessment, 26
Service delivery
    follow-up in, 128
    stepped-care model, 127–128
Service integration, 123–131
    alcohol screening role in, 126–
        127
    broad-based model for, 126
    continuum of, 126
    training suggestions, 125–126
Sexual assault, 8
Sexual risk taking, 8
Skills-building exercises, 89
Sleep interruptions, 9
"Slips," 83, 99
Smoking, survey data, 8
Sociability, as risk factor, 15
Social Context of Drinking Scale,
    38
"Social loafing," in groups, 110
Socialization processes, 15–16
Sociocultural model, 14
Sorority membership, 16
Stages-of-change model
    intervention implications, 19–
        20
    overview, 17–19
Standard drink, definition, 28

"Stepped-care" model
    follow-up requirement, 128
    in service delivery, 127–128
Strategies for Low-Risk Drinking,
    197–198
    example of use of, 98
    and group problem solving, 120
    and readiness for change, 81
Stress, as risk factor, 15, 17
Structured Clinical Interview for
    DSM-IV, 34
Student opinions/perceptions, 10–11
Summaries, 55–57
    in closing a session, 78–79
    definition, 55
    functions of, 56–57

Time Line Follow-Back, 30, 40
Traffic accidents, 8
Training, 128–130
    brief interventions, 128–129
    group interventions, 129
    longer interventions, 129
    practice and feedback in, 129–
        130
    and service integration, 125–126
Transtheoretical model of change
    intervention implications, 19–20
    overview, 17–19
"Triggers," in functional analysis
    exercise, 89–90

TWEAK questionnaire, 35
Two group facilitators. See Co-
    leader teams

Universal prevention, 124

Values Cards, 91, 118, 171–178
Values cardsort exercise, 171–178
    discrepancy-building method,
        groups, 109, 118
    example of use of, 99
    in groups, 118
    life values identification, 91–93
Values clarification programs, 21–22
Videotaped training
    demonstrations, 129
Violence, 9
"Volume–variability" index, 29

Web-based feedback, 86
Women, heavy drinking
    prevalence, 2–3, 5
Workshops, in training skills, 129

Young Adult Alcohol Problems
    Screening Test (YAAPST),
        138–140
    feedback function, 86–87
    negative consequences
        assessment, 32–33, 40
    time constraints, 96